THE VIRUS KILLER

Books by Irwin Philip Sobel

THE VIRUS KILLER
THE HOSPITAL MAKERS

THE
VIRUS
KILLER

Irwin Philip Sobel

Doubleday & Company, Inc.
GARDEN CITY, NEW YORK, 1975

Library of Congress Cataloging in Publication Data
Sobel, Irwin Philip.
The virus killer.
I. Title. [DNLM: 1. Interferon—Popular works.
QW800 S677v]
PZ4.S676Vi [PS3569.02]   813'.5'4
ISBN 0-385-09563-5
Library of Congress Catalog Card Number 74-24715

To Margaret and Michael
and the old friends,
Abe Abeloff
Artie Cracovaner
Sam Handelman
Marty Jacobs
Johnnie Kilroe
Mac Nurnberg
Julian Rogatz
Henry Sarason

THE VIRUS KILLER

1

FOR YEARS everyone in the Department of Virology had been saying that he was peculiar. He had no friends, never courted a girl, answered questions in grunts and monosyllables, and broke out in a silly smile at the most inappropriate times. But Dr. Choate defended him. "He keeps his mouth shut and works hard. What more do you want of a technician?" This October morning, the silly smile unaccountably present, he listened without response to his chief's telephone summons. Then he stood up, lit a rose-tipped Reemstma-Senoussi, and after inhaling once, threw the burning cigarette out the tenth-story window. He entered the office without knocking, and although a member of the board of trustees of the Medical Center was seated across the desk from his chief, he made no apology. Dr. Choate frowned, but all he said was,

"How much of the interferon solution do we have left?"

"Twenty ml."

"Bring it to me before you go to lunch. Dr. Keats is picking it up at two this afternoon, and he's as punctual as sunrise."

"Sunset would suit him better," the technician said and walked out.

"Is it customary for the help to comment on the careers of doctors?" asked the trustee.

The chief of Virology shrugged. "That was just a puff of steam from a hidden volcano. As a matter of fact he likes Keats. He thinks the world has given him a raw deal."

"Tell me about this doctor who is walking into the twilight."

"He's a former classmate of mine, a top-flight pediatrician who has never hit the jackpot. To be a success a good medical man has to be a good medicine man. I'm afraid Jim Keats never bothered with the feathers, the rattles, and the tom-toms. His hospital is John Quincy Adams, where research is tabu. There, after he sees his patients, he putters around in a little half-assed laboratory of his own and is ignored."

To Choate's surprise the old man replied, "Half an ass is better than none. Now tell me what interferon is."

"A virus multiplies only inside body cells. Interferon will sometimes prevent it from growing there. When it comes to repelling a serious viral infection, though, it's just another Maginot Line. And it doesn't cure anything."

"Then why did I give you four hundred thousand dollars last year?"

Choate laughed. "We do a few other things besides working with interferon. You gave me the money because you're a frustrated scientist and love the Medical Center. And because you know that we live in a viral age. Polio, smallpox, mumps, measles, and chickenpox are all caused by viruses. So are influenza, rabies, and the common cold. From hepatitis, an inflammation of the liver, to encephalitis, an inflammation of the brain, you're traveling along the viral road. Sure, we can prevent the occurrence of viral diseases with wonderful new vaccines. And we can successfully treat more and more germ diseases with penicillin and other antibiotics. But there isn't an antibiotic in the world that has the slightest effect on a virus. Any doctor who tells you that he cures viral diseases with penicillin is conning you. There is no such thing as a virus killer."

"If you release that to the press, there will be wailing in the suburbs. People with colds and flu line up there for penicillin shots the way people in Manhattan do for three-and-a-half-dollar movies."

"My findings appear only in the scientific literature."

"Do you think you will ever come up with a virus killer?"

Choate shook his head. "I'm fifty-four. In ten and a half years they will throw me out. Oh, I know that because of my papers on tissue culture and my monograph on the causal relationship between the Epstein Barr virus and infectious mononucleosis they may keep me on an extra six months. But there just isn't enough time."

The old man crossed his legs. "Philanthropist trustees are more fortunate. They have relative immortality. I am seventy-five, and no one on the board would dare to remind me of it. Only God can make me resign, and He calls it death. There is no mandatory retirement age for giving away money. Did you ever hear of an institution refusing a million-dollar gift because the donor was over sixty-five?"

He looked around the room with distaste. Cardboard crates filled with new equipment lay haphazardly on the threadbare carpet as if an attempt were being made to trip the unwary. Beautifully bound, gilt-labeled sets of medical periodicals rested in dilapidated wooden bookcases like golden girls in the arms of tattered lovers. The top of the cheap metal desk was concealed by manuscripts, microscope slides, and a large blotter that looked as if it were the first one manufactured when the use of sand was discontinued.

"When you make up your budget in December," the trustee continued, "you can count on me for another four hundred thousand dollars," he raised his hand to forestall any thanks, "provided that you refurnish this office. It's a disgrace to the Medical Center."

Choate looked at him appealingly. "I like to put every penny I get into research."

The old man sighed. "But can't you find a more suitable ashtray than that urinal you have on top of your desk? You can buy a less unorthodox one in Woolworth's for forty-nine cents."

"All right. I'll refurnish my office with a new ashtray. Agreed?"

The old man nodded, rose, and walked to the door. The chief of Virology followed him.

"I don't know what my department would do without you."

The old man said nothing until he reached the door. Then he turned. "I don't know what I would do without your department. It's given me the urge to live."

The fact that the technician had been seen leaving the departmental office removed any suspicion from what he later did. Those of his strange actions which were noticed by his coworkers were interpreted as the results of his chief's commands. First he carried the flask of interferon he had just removed from the refrigerator to the positive-pressure room. Working under the laminar flow hood, where a curtain of sterile air kept out all contaminants, he poured it into a small bottle just as Dr. Choate had requested. Then he dumped most of it down the sink. The silly smile fluttered. He made sucking noises like a baby at the breast. Oh, Dr. Keats would get his twenty ml. all right, he said to himself, but when he did it would not be that silly old interferon alone, but a combination of wonderful things. He walked down to the ninth floor and returned with a tube of tobacco mosaic virus, a little of which he pipetted into the bottle. In the next half hour two other plant viruses and three animal viruses went into the mixture. Bacteriophage, IDU, and amantidine proved irresistible. These too were carried into the positive-pressure room. Growing more confident, he took the elevator to the sixth floor, where he removed some reverse transcriptase from the Department of Enzymology. In the biochemistry laboratories he found four types of RNA and three of DNA particularly appealing. He was not greedy. He used only small amounts. Everything he handled he carefully replaced. No one would ever know what he had touched. Under the hood his technique was impeccable. The necks of the vessels were flamed in a Bunsen burner both before and after each procedure. Although the other technicians worked with bare hands, he used sterile plastic gloves for every transfer. When the bottle in the positive-pressure room was filled at noon, there were thirty-six pairs of discarded gloves in the trash basket. He flamed the neck for the last time and then stirred the fluid with a glass rod, murmuring, "Mix, mix, mix, mix." By this time he had completely forgotten what he had put in the bottle.

He took it to the subbasement, where the Department of Radiology kept the big linear accelerator in a lead-lined room. A faded old woman with little hair, beady eyes, and a face like a chicken barred his way.

He held up the bottle. "Professor Choate wants this irradiated with five thousand rads."

The X-ray supervisor looked as if she were about to have her chicken neck cut. "Five thousand rads! That will take thirty minutes."

A tough-looking attending with five o'clock shadow and five children at home to further prove his virility walked up to them. "What the professor wants the professor gets," he said to the woman. He turned to the technician. "This machine handles six million electron volts. It's death on the sex organs." He peered into the distance. "See that room at the end of the corridor? Sit there for half an hour. You don't look as if you have much testicular reserve."

The technician flushed and walked away.

At one o'clock he was in Dr. Choate's office. "Here's the interferon solution you asked for," he mumbled. The silly smile flashed as he put the bottle in a small refrigerator near the desk.

At two o'clock Keats knocked on the door and walked in.

"The usual Count of Monte Cristo punctuality," said the virologist, rising. He saw the watery eyes and red nose, and heard the cough. "A present from your little patients?"

Keats nodded and sat down on the chair near the desk. "I appreciate your letting me have the interferon, Bill."

"It's no big deal. I've reached the end of the road with interferon. It's no longer scientifically profitable for me to go ahead with it. I did read a clinical article in this week's *Lancet,* though, that might interest you. Naturally, the *New York Times* ran a summary the week before. Investigators in Salisbury, England, dropped rhinovirus type four into the noses of a control group of volunteers. That's one of the two-hundred-odd viruses that cause the common cold. They sprayed the insides of the noses of a second group with massive amounts of interferon both before and after the application of rhino four. The symptoms of the common cold were less severe in this group than in the controls. Nothing too exciting, but I thought you might like to repeat this work on children. If you can persuade the John Quincy Adams stuffed shirts to let you perform the experiment, I'll let you have some rhinovirus four. Of course, don't inject the interferon intravenously."

"They aren't very receptive to new ideas, but I'll try." He blew his nose and coughed. "You're the fair-haired boy up here now. I appreciate the boosts you've given me down through the years."

"Cut the crap, Jim. I still envy you for the way you used to run the off-tackle slant for Columbia."

Keats patted his belly. "You're not the only one. I envy the way I used to do it myself. But you're all-American now, Bill. I hear you were considered for the Nobel Prize in Medicine last year."

"Sure, sure, I was considered all right." He moved some papers from one side of the desk to another. "Fifty years ago my grandfather was on the Swedish Nobel Prize Committee. He was a heller. He had two friends on the committee who were hellers, too. At the time there was a woman called Birgit something-or-other who was famous all over Stockholm. She was a leader of the peace movement. But that's not why she was famous. There were no wars going on anywhere at the time. She was famous because of her chastity. A handsome, voluptuous-looking spinster of forty, she looked askance at even platonic friendships. Who knew what they might lead to? Any man who grasped her elbow to help her across the street she regarded as a potential rapist and showed it with a devastating glance. Hand kissing she abhorred. Many a heel-clicking German was left grasping empty air as he bowed and murmured, *'Küss die Hand, gnädiges*

Fräulein.' Her purity was so well publicized that it became legendary throughout the city. A grocer holding up a bottle of mineral water before a stubborn customer would often say, 'It's as pure as Birgit,' to clinch the sale. One Sunday afternoon my grandfather and his two friends, pores oozing aquavite, were chatting with a government minister at their club. Her name came up. My grandfather and his two cynical friends fully agreed with George Bernard Shaw's definition of virtue, which was 'insufficient temptation.' They bet the minister one hundred kronen that within a month each of them would have slept with the beautiful Birgit. The rules were strict. All three had to possess her, as they would have said in those days. So confident were they that they gave their opponent odds of two to one. Their confidence proved justified. They all laid her within a week. Their seduction technique was simple and aboveboard. Each promised to consider her for the Nobel Peace Prize. When it was over they kept their word. They *did* consider her. Only they never discussed their thoughts with anyone else. In the end everyone was satisfied, the friends because they had won their bet, Birgit because she knew she had been considered for the Nobel Prize, and the lecherous minister because he enjoyed the descriptions of the three nights of love his opponents so generously gave him. Of the five, my grandfather came out the worst. A drawing of straws forced him to tackle her first. She was a virgin with a calcified hymen. His penis took a terrible beating while her vagina seemed insensitive. The following week he always remembered as one of the worst in his life. My grandmother was a very demanding woman once they went to bed. That week she happened to be more demanding than ever. Such were the wages of sin." He tapped his cigarette ash into the urinal on his desk and smiled bitterly. "They considered me for the Nobel Prize last year as seriously as they once considered Birgit."

"And they screwed you as thoroughly, too. Bill, you're the Nobelist virologist of them all."

Choate reached into the drawer, took out a metal box the size of a sugar cube, and stood up. He was six foot six.

"What's that?" asked Keats.

"It's a tape recorder I once built," answered Choate.

He lifted the top for a moment, revealing a tape as thin as sewing thread. "Press the wire," he said as he handed the instrument to his friend.

Keats pushed down the thin wire release. Immediately an incredibly clear and tiny voice came from the cube he was now holding carefully between his thumb and index finger. Choate took it from him, shut it off, and put it back in his desk. He sat down slowly.

"It's Willem van der Noot's acceptance speech in Stockholm. He was the Nobel Prize winner in Medicine last year."

People first noticed how big Bill Choate was when he began to walk at ten months. The faster he grew the more he prized little things. At an age when most children wanted to go to the zoo to see the lions, tigers, and elephants, he was fascinated by insects. It was the dwarf, not the giant, in the fairy tales who held his attention. When he was twelve he discovered that boats could be built inside bottles. He constructed a scale model of the U.S.S. *Constitution* in a small, burnt-out bulb his mother had used as a night light. She told her friends that she was sure his secret ambition was to engrave the Lord's prayer on the head of a pin. When he was fourteen his father offered to buy him a ten-speed English bicycle. He asked for a microscope instead. In medical school he resolved to devote his free time to the study of the smallest living objects which were emphasized in the curriculum. They proved to be germs. He haunted the bacteriology laboratories.

As soon as he received his M.D. he went to the Massachusetts Institute of Technology to learn something about the smallest particles in the universe, the electron and the atomic nucleus. In four years he received a Ph.D. in atomic physics. But he became dissatisfied with inanimate objects. After all, he was a physician. Since bacteria had proved too big for his liking, he decided to devote the rest of his career to the study of viruses, the smallest of all living organisms. For three years he worked at the Rockefeller Institute with Dr. Thomas Rivers, the eminent virologist. Then he went to the Medical Center. The discovery of the electron microscope gave a tremendous boost to his career. Viruses are too small to be seen under even the most powerful light microscope. They are, however, easily visible under the electron microscope. Choate's knowledge of atomic physics enabled him to make important contributions to the development of the newer instrument. By 1973 he was recognized as one of the greatest virologists in the world. But the Nobel Prize, which he felt he deserved, had never been offered to him. He consoled himself with the thought that although Karl Landsteiner had discovered the blood groups in 1901, a feat that made blood transfusions possible, he did not become a Nobelist until 1930.

Choate had met and become fond of Keats in medical school. Fame had not interfered with the relationship. He liked his old friends to be big. The submicroscopic viruses which had killed so many millions, though fascinating, he came to regard as enemies.

"I hear your chief at Adams is retiring in a couple of months," he said to Keats. "Are they going to give you the shaft?"

Keats shrugged. "I don't know. Three years ago they brought in a thirty-five-year-old kid who had just finished his training. There's talk that they're grooming him to be the next director of Pediatrics." He blew his nose. "I'm afraid that thirty years of service to the hospital have just made me old and familiar."

"You harp on your age too much. I don't mean to be offensive, but I think it's largely your wife's fault. Rubens, the painter, had the right philosophy. When he was sixty he fell in love with a girl of sixteen. Not only that, but he decided to marry her. His friends were appalled. Finally one of them said, 'Peter Paul, do you realize that when you are seventy-four she will be thirty?' The old man thought this over for a while. Then he replied, 'Well, if that day ever comes, I'll get myself another sixteen-year-old girl.' With that spirit, Jim, you can go out and lick the world."

He walked to the icebox, took out the bottle, and held it up to the window. "It's as good as the stuff the Salisbury group used. I'll bet it cost us five thousand dollars to make what's in here. I don't know whether you can do anything with it. I don't even know whether you will get a paper out of it. But one thing I guarantee. This interferon is pure."

When Keats reached the street he found that a twenty-five-dollar ticket had been placed on the windshield of his car. His MD license plate, as usual, had not protected him. He made a quick calculation. His trip to the Medical Center had cost him more than one third of his net income for the day. True, he earned six or seven thousand dollars a year more than a garbage collector. But not much more than a police sergeant. He got into his 1966 Ford and drove to John Quincy Adams Hospital with the bottle carefully cradled in the inside pocket of his jacket directly over his heart. He coughed all the way there.

At exactly three o'clock the technician at the Medical Center began opening the cabinets in the main virology laboratory and throwing the glassware on the floor. Soon he was hurling petri dishes, flasks, bottles, and tubes against the ceiling. He never aimed at anyone, and the technicians standing quietly against the walls were not about to find out whether he would if they advanced upon him. When the police arrived he was overturning the microscopes. At the sight of the sergeant and the three patrolmen he stood rigidly at attention. And he did not say a word while he was being frisked until he felt a hand patting the inside of his thighs. Then he murmured, "You're a nice man." It was at this moment that Professor Choate walked in. He quickly assessed the damages at over a thousand dollars. To the policeman who approached notebook in hand he said, "No charges will be preferred against this man. Just take him across the street, gently." Then he left.

The technician assumed the at-ease position. "Before I leave you do you mind if I recite a poem I once wrote?" he asked.

The policemen's expressions did not change.

He picked up a pair of sterile gloves from the worktable, drew them on expertly, and plucked a piece of paper from his pocket. Then he intoned,

"Mix them together
    Rocks and heather,
    Day and night,
    Black and white,
    Bricks and mortar
    Son and daughter.
    Then whip them with a thousand sticks
    Till men grow breasts and women pricks."

The policemen applauded halfheartedly.
"Deep."
"Elegant."
"Lots of pizzaz."
"I got a friend who's an expert on poems," said the sergeant. "How about reading it to him?"

The technician raised his head and walked stiffly to the door. It was in the elevator that it began. First softly, then more loudly he barked, "Mix, mix, mix, MIX!" over and over again. Once in the

18

street the police enclosed him in a hollow square and marched across the plaza to the rhythm of his cadences. The oldest of the patrolmen, a veteran of World War II, felt as if he were plodding on tired feet to the "Hup, hoop, heep, HAWP!" of his drillmaster at Fort Devon. They entered the psychiatric hospital in perfect step. There was no trouble.

At a quarter to six that evening Professor Choate received a telephone call from the chief psychiatric resident.

"Your technician is a paranoid schizophrenic, suh. The outlook is very bad. So far we haven't been able to make much contact with him. Most of the time he sits on his bed muttering, 'Mix, mix, mix, MIX.'" There was a long pause. Then the soft drawl returned. "He's not some kind of an integrationist, is he, suh?"

Choate assured the resident that he was not.

2

JOHN QUINCY ADAMS Hospital occupied an entire city block in the heart of New York's fashionable upper East Side. Its primary concern was the treatment of patients. Research was not encouraged, but since a six-hundred-bed institution was supposed to keep up with the times, a few rooms on the top of an old building scheduled for early demolition were reserved for those of its doctors who wished to conduct scientific experiments. Just as a private school in the twenties might have admitted a single Negro pupil to show that it was free of prejudice, so half a century later Adams accepted the idea of token research to show that it was free of backwardness. Grants were rarely obtained since the caliber of the investigations did not attract them. Over a twenty-five-year period Keats had received only two, one from the government and one from a private donor. As he entered his top floor laboratory room he was worrying about a dog who had survived blood-volume determinations as an experimental animal only to be struck down by a lethal attack of distemper as a pet.

It lay on a blanket, eyes filled with pus, nose encrusted with a brown exudate, breathing rapidly from fever and pneumonia. On the floor next to it were vomitus and a diarrheal stool. Keats placed the bottle from the Medical Center in the small refrigerator. He took off his jacket, put on his workcoat, and cleaned up the mess with wet paper towels. When he whistled, the mongrel came toward him dragging its hind legs. They were completely paralyzed. He put it back on its blanket. Then he sat on a wooden chair to keep it company while it died. It was too bad nothing more could be done, he reflected. Well, it wasn't his responsibility. The animal belonged to everybody, to the doctors, the technicians, the porters, the cleaning women, to all the people who worked in this piss-pot excuse for a research lab. He had done everything he could. He had called in a veterinarian who had charged more than he himself did for a house call. Just before the man left he had expressed surprise that no preventive injections had been given.

Keats walked to the bookcase and pulled out Topley and Wilson's microbiology. Yes, distemper was caused by a virus, a myxovirus related to the ones that caused mumps and influenza. He replaced the book and sat down again, wondering whether the weak antiviral substance he had just received would help the poor animal. In a second he realized that the thought was absurd. Interferon was species specific. Only dog interferon was suitable in this case. What Choate had handed him was human interferon made from the white cells of blood donors. So what harm could come of giving a little of the stuff to the dying dog? he asked himself. Come to think of it, what was he going to do with the five-thousand-dollar genie in the bottle? To seriously consider a pediatric repetition of the Salisbury experiment would be suicidal. Research on human beings was tabu at Adams. And anyone who in the opinion of the medical board was interested in making guinea pigs out of children would be considered depraved. Soon he would have to put in his application for the directorship of Pediatrics. A formal request for permission to start an interferon investigation at Adams would destroy whatever chance of success he might otherwise have. Bill Choate meant well, but he never understood the difference between a voluntary and a university hospital.

The Medical Center had three times as many beds as Adams. Although its patients received good care, the larger institution was oriented toward research, the training of residents, and the teaching of the students in its medical school. Tens of millions of dollars had been spent on building its laboratories and stocking them with the most modern and sophisticated equipment. If a physician wanted to remain on the staff, he had to write articles which were published in the better scientific periodicals, read papers before medical conventions, and act as a panelist on key programs throughout the country. The experiments on which his reputation rested were very expensive. At Adams, on the other hand, research was frowned upon, for one thing, because it was so costly. The only money that could be raised was for new buildings. Its residents were in the main a facade which permitted it to qualify as a teaching institution. And there was no university to back it in difficult times. Finally, the doctors at the Medical Center were full time, that is they were salaried employees. The members of the medical staff were not private practitioners as they were at Adams.

Keats realized that he should never have accepted the gift.

But now that he had it what was he going to do with it? Rub it on his thinning hair? Pour it over his penis in the hope that Annie Laurie would go to bed with him again after three years? Maybe he ought to take it to Salisbury and squirt it up Oswald Moseley's fascist ass. But Moseley was probably dead.

He went to the refrigerator, took out the bottle, and removed one ml. of the fluid with a sterile, disposable syringe which he then placed together with an alcohol-soaked cottonball on one end of the metal worktable. After a long pause he picked up the dog. As soon as he did the twitchings began. These he diagnosed as manifestations of encephalitis, an inflammation of the brain caused by distemper virus. He laid the animal on the table, reaching for the syringe with his right hand. During an interval between convulsions he used his left hand as a tourniquet, squeezing a foreleg close to the body. The vein became prominent at once. It was now easy to insert the needle, and, after releasing the pressure exerted by his left hand, to empty the contents of the syringe into the vessel. Then he removed the injection unit. The entire procedure had taken twenty seconds.

He laid the dog on its blanket, poured fresh water into the dish near its head, took off his workcoat, and, after scrubbing his hands meticulously, put on his jacket. By the time he reached the door the seizures had ceased. The animal was breathing slowly. It looked a little better but he decided that he was indulging in a wish-fulfillment fantasy.

He crossed the bridge to the main building, which housed the Department of Pediatrics and its small lecture room, where he was about to give a talk to the residents. Thirty years before he had joined the house staff as an intern. But there were no interns now. Only residents. Nobody entered the Army as a private anymore. Everyone came in as a sergeant. In 1922, the year Adams was founded, members of the house staff were given a room and food but no salary. It would never have occurred to them to ask for one. The medical schools had not paid them. On the contrary, their parents had to pay these institutions a yearly tuition fee. Hospital training was obviously an extension of medical school. The young interns of the past were delighted that this important part of their education was free. In the late thirties pressure from the residents forced Adams to pay them a small salary. Today, a first-year man was given twelve thousand dollars a year. In his fourth year he received eighteen and demanded twenty. Two thirds of the graduating classes in the medical schools were married, often to fellow students. After such couples entered Adams, the family income eventually reached thirty-six thousand dollars a year at a time when they had neither finished their postgraduate training nor treated a patient of their own. The forty-hour week was quite generally observed except by the few whose atavism made them put in a few hours more. In their final year those residents attached to the Department of Pediatrics were allowed a three-month observation tour of any children's hospital of their choice, even in Paris, London, Amsterdam, or Tel Aviv. This was in addition to their regular month's vacation. Couples were therefore being paid thirty-six thousand dollars for eight months' work. Interestingly enough, as the residents' salaries increased, so did their reputation for idealism.

On television, hospital dramas were replacing Westerns. The screen's chief resident had become a composite of the square-shooting marshal and the good Indian. If the real Indians had done one tenth as well as the real residents, there would have been no confrontation at Wounded Knee.

Unfortunately, the quality of the house staff had deteriorated over the past twenty years. One irritable old attending had invented the Ab/Co ratio to measure the decline. In this equation Ab equaled ability, Co cockiness. He claimed that a generation ago Ab over Co equaled twenty. Today, he said, it was one twentieth. This was nonsense, of course, but the ratio had changed.

As Keats approached the main building he was trying to figure out why the residents he was about to address, as well as all the others, were so cosseted by the hospital. The youngsters coming out of Adams's womb were being smothered in the pubic hair of maternal indulgence. He smiled. Maybe it was because they were unique. A doctor could be wise a thousand times during a long lifetime, but young only once.

The members of the house staff had for their part given him a special dispensation. Attendings of his age, they felt, should properly restrict their lectures to clinical topics and bedside medicine. He, on the other hand, knew that they would be exposed to these practical aspects of their specialty for the rest of their careers in private practice. Their residencies offered them the last chance to learn something about chemistry, physics, physiology, and microbiology. His carefully prepared talks were, therefore, devoted for the most part to the basic sciences. It had not taken the young doctors long to realize that he was doing what was best for them.

He began, "If a man who has lived a sedentary existence takes up jogging, he must expect his legs to hurt. That is because he is using muscles he never used before. If you concentrate on what I am saying, you will soon get a headache. That is because you will be using your brain, an organ on which you have heretofore been careful not to make excessive demands."

His topic was blood-group immunology with emphasis on the technique of exchange transfusion, a procedure he had introduced at the hospital twenty-four years before. In it, a newborn baby's blood is almost completely removed and replaced with donor blood. At the end, the young audience applauded.

Since he had found a legal parking place near the hospital, he walked to his office on Park Avenue and Eighty-fourth Street. It consisted of a very small waiting room, an even smaller consulting room, and a tiny examining room. The entire suite was not much bigger than the average living room. But then his patients were not very big either, he reasoned. For this he paid five thousand dollars a year. His malpractice insurance was more than ten times as much as it had once been. Expenses were high, income low.

He sat at his desk blowing his nose for what he estimated was the hundredth time, and glanced at his mail. The doorman, a compassionate fellow, always placed the checks on top. Keats wondered whether he candled the envelopes. This afternoon there were no checks to balance the bills mixed with the advertisements. The telephone rang six times. There were two cancellations of appointments, one wrong number, and three requests by mothers that he fill out immediately the school forms they had received two months before and mailed to him yesterday. It seemed as if he heard nothing pleasant over the telephone anymore. He knew exactly what would happen if he bought a ticket for the million-dollar lottery. One day his part-time secretary would rush into his consultation room, cheeks flushed, eyes aglow, screaming, "The director of the lottery is on the line." He would pick up the receiver and hear the unctuous voice say, "This is Nelson B. Throwdyce, Director of Lotteries of the state of New York. We have just completed the drawing and I want you to know," here there would be a long pause, "that you lost." Oh, well, maybe it was his cold that was making him so irritable. He wondered whether it had gone to his sinuses.

He picked up a letter from the pile. It was from the John Quincy Adams Ladies Aid Society, urging him to buy two tickets to a musical comedy benefit at fifty dollars each. For a hundred dollars he could buy a dress for Annie Laurie, he said to himself. Not that he had bought her any clothes in the past two years. Inflation had robbed him of his good intentions. Besides, pediatrics was dead in Manhattan. The middle-class and the rich, at least those of childbearing age, were moving away. Obstetrics, which provided the life-blood of his specialty with an unending stream of newborns, was dying too. Formerly most pregnant women who lived in the suburbs were delivered in Manhattan. Now they had their babies in surburban hospitals. The older Adams obstetricians, those who had once fed him cases, did no more obstetrics and were concentrating on gynecology. As one of them said, "A man doesn't give up obstetrics. Obstetrics gives up the man."

Keats read through the October issue of the *American Journal of Diseases of Children* and then went home. It took him fifty minutes to find a legal parking place. He considered himself lucky. Annie Laurie was unloading her supermarket purchases from a cart. The hundred and ten dollars a week he gave her did not go very far these days, he realized. As usual, she looked angry.

"Rough day at the office?" he asked.

"Well, I didn't sit on my ass the way you did. You think it's easy for a woman of my age to hold down a full-time job and then come home and run a house. First I have to do the marketing, then the cooking, then the dishes while you're reading your books or looking at television. And who do you think does the laundry? That stupid cleaning woman who comes in once a week? It takes her two hours to iron a handkerchief. All right, so I've got a washing machine and a dishwasher, and you take the shirts out to the Chinaman. Big provider! But I'm putting in a twelve-hour day. What kind of life is that for a woman?"

She continued to sort the groceries. He blew his nose. She turned to him. "Will you please use Kleenexes instead of handkerchiefs? Do you expect me to wash those filthy, infected things? And while we're on the subject, I've told you a thousand times to turn your socks inside out when you take them off."

He looked at her. She was still beautiful. Why shouldn't she be? he asked himself. She was only thirty-eight.

His first wife, the daughter of an eminent American conductor and herself a pianist of almost concert caliber, had been warm, tender, and loving. But quite homely, he was forced to admit. Only her breasts had been beautiful. When the cancer struck, it lodged in the left one as if to show that no beauty could stand up to it. He walked alongside the stretcher as they wheeled her to the operating room. When they reached the elevator, she pulled his head down to her lips, placed his hand on the breast, and whispered, "Love it a little for the last time." The breast and the armpit lymph glands were carefully removed. It was a very good job. One year later the malignant growth had spread to the lungs and bones. A year after that she was dead. He often wondered whether he could have saved her life if he had noticed the little lump while they were making love. Then he would try to think of something else.

Four years after her death he met Annie Laurie. Her icy sexuality had attracted and then repelled more than one lover. There had been no prolonged relationships. A member of a poor family in Flushing, she had worked as a night waitress to put herself through secretarial school. When he first saw her, she was a typist in the Adams record room, twenty-eight, and at the height of her beauty. She helped him find a chart which had eluded the other girls for two days and loaned him her ballpoint pen since he had forgotten to transfer his from his jacket to his white coat. On the way out fifteen minutes later he leaned over her desk and said,

"I wonder whether you would have dinner with me tonight."

"I'm wondering, too. I wonder why an important Park Avenue doctor would want to take a record-room typist out to dinner." She looked up at him shrewdly. "Are you married?"

"My wife is dead."

That evening he took her to the Carlyle. It was a very expensive meal. She was astounded that neither at dinner nor during the long ride to Queens did he attempt to seduce her. She was alone in her one-room apartment at ten. After that he took her out two or three times a week, to the theater, the opera, concerts, and football games. She had two qualities he admired—a good ear for music and the ability to chat. Silence, he felt, was masculine. And she was lovely over every square inch of her body, he was sure. A cancer would have to strike at too many places to ever totally destroy her beauty. Three months after they had met they went to his apartment one night and made love. Or rather he made love. She was quite passive. But she eventually responded in a controlled sort of way and even had a muted orgasm.

Soon she was sure that he would ask her to marry him. Her friends in the record room looked up his age in the Directory of Medical Specialists. One of them said to her,

"Do you think you're being smart? He is sixteen years older than you."

Her reply was, "I know, but he's very well preserved."

He was forty-four.

She found him interesting and unusual. She had never gone out with a doctor. At Adams, residents and young attendings dated, slept with, and often married nurses, but never girls from the record room. Her inquiries revealed that he was considered to be the best pediatrician in the hospital. From childhood she had been led to believe that a good doctor made money. If he did not, the dictum ran, he was not a good doctor. Keats, she decided, could give her the only thing she had ever wanted from a man—security. It was not that she was mercenary. It was simply that none of her family had ever had security. And she had seen what had happened to them.

They were married by a justice of the peace. For the first five years they both were satisfied with the arrangement. She gave up her job at once. As a result of door-to-door stops and the following up of every lead in the *New York Times,* she found a pleasant, inexpensive, four-room rent-controlled apartment on the East Side. She was impressed by his friends. Later she became quite comfortable in their presence. The lack of a college education she tried to compensate for by taking courses at the New School, reading extensively, and visiting museums and art galleries. She became a good cook and had always been a good housekeeper. His income, though small, reached a peak and stayed there. They took a month's vacation every year and once spent five weeks in Europe. Sexual intercourse was regular, and if not passionate, at least adequate.

Then, after five years, his practice began to slip away. He found himself losing patients faster than he could replace them. Young couples with children were leaving for the suburbs in increasing numbers. Young executives with families were being told by the front office to report to Atlanta, Des Moines, Duluth, or even London. Gypsy America was on the march. Older obstetricians, having gone over to the practice of gynecology, were no longer interested in taking care of the dwindling number of pregnant Manhattanites and the irregular hours such a task would entail. Their younger colleagues sent what newborns they could to pediatricians of their own age. Annie Laurie suddenly realized that Jim had never been and would never be a money maker. As his income diminished so did her dreams of security.

They had always slept in one bed. Now she began to complain that his tossing disturbed her and that his nightly trip to the toilet kept her awake.

"There must be something wrong with your prostate," she said to him. "You should have it removed."

He bought twin beds, and gave their old one to the Salvation Army. But she found a greater irritation. He was beginning to snore. She told him to lie on his side or his chest. It did no good. He evidently would have snored if he had slept standing on his head, she at last decided. When she could stand it no longer, she had the dining room set moved into the living room. Her own bed and bureau replaced it. She kept her door closed at night. More and more frequently she rejected his advances, first with the standard polite excuses, headache, fatigue, or just-not-in-the-mood, then with a curt "no."

In 1971 his financial position began to deteriorate rapidly, squeezed as he now was between the onset of inflation and the dwindling income caused by the exodus of his patients. He paid the rent, and took care of the utilities and the major expenses. But the weekly allowance he gave her did little more than pay for the food. And there were her clothes, shoes, cosmetics, hair dressing and dental bills, as well as house refurbishing and countless incidentals. Worst of all, there were no stocks or bonds, and little money in the bank. She decided that she would have to take a job. She found one at once as office manager for an insurance company. An excellent salary reinforced her determination to put something away for her old age. She resolved not to end up like her mother.

The first day she arrived at work a half hour early. That night he asked her whether she would like to make love.

"Give it up," she answered. "You're too old."

He never touched her again.

She hated having to work; she hated her job; and she hated the idea of having a husband who could not support her.

He watched her unpack the groceries. She was still a beautiful woman, he had to admit.

He took *Gravity's Rainbow* to the toilet and read one page as he did every evening. He figured that he would be able to finish it in two years. If he became constipated, he would do it in one. At dinner, which they ate in the kitchen, Annie Laurie was as chatty as ever. She had not, he reflected, lost that gift. Only now her conversation, once so lively, was restricted to the annoyances that had beset her at the office. He nodded but said nothing. What should he tell her? That he had tried to save a dog's life that afternoon? Once during the meal he saw her searching for the saltcellar. He lifted it and was about to hand it to her, but she said,

"Put it down! You know I can't stand having you touch anything with those disgusting warts on the back of your hand. I've asked you over and over again to have them removed, but you never do anything I say."

After she put away the dishes, they sat in the living room reading the papers. Suddenly she exclaimed,

"Will you stop that constant snuffling! It drives me up the wall. I know why you do it—just to annoy me."

Several times he tried to clear his throat as quietly as he could, but she rustled the papers ominously at each attempt. In the end, listening to his cough proved too much for her. She picked up her book, walked stiffly to her room, and closed the door. At ten-thirty he went to bed. As he lay on his back trying to sleep, he realized that at his age it was too late for another start. His death, not divorce, would end the marriage. In the meantime he was going to avoid fighting with her at any cost. As he fell asleep he remembered the dog. He would have to get up early to give it an ashcan funeral.

He awakened at seven with a headache and a sore throat. When he threw off the covers and sat up, he felt chilly, a sure sign, he knew, that he had fever. He took his temperature by mouth while he was dressing. It was one hundred and two. He had always been possessed by an irrational fear that if he did not show up for work for a few days, he would starve. There was no one to mind the store, he reasoned. He had a wordless breakfast with Annie Laurie, retreating once to his bedroom when he felt a fit of coughing coming on. He must avoid anything which would irritate her.

Parking in the shadow of John Quincy Adams Hospital gave him no protection against a twenty-five-dollar fine, he knew. Though the police disliked the idea of harassing doctors, they were forced to do so in their unwilling role of city tax collectors. A patrolman could easily bring in a thousand dollars a day for New York simply by getting rid of forty tickets during his tour of duty. Attitudes toward doctors had changed in a generation. Keats's father, a hard-working pediatrician, could have parked illegally in front of a whorehouse if he had wanted to. Any member of the force so callous as to take a sheaf of summonses from his pocket would have been surrounded by a hostile mob which, through a spokesman, a devout old lady as likely as not, would have shouted, "You let the doctor alone, do you hear! He needs a bit of relaxation now and then." Today, the people enjoyed the discomfiture of physicians. Special privileges were no longer automatically conferred. Repeatedly the laity said, "The trouble is that the wives take advantage of the MD license plate," forgetting perhaps the number of women who practiced medicine in town.

When Keats reached the corridor leading to his little laboratory he had a slight chill due, he felt, either to his infection or to the idea of having to dispose of the dog's body. At least his cold would protect him from the smell. He opened the door reluctantly. The animal was standing in the middle of the room, eyes clear, respiration slow, nose moist and free of pus, and hind legs firm. There was no paralysis. He closed the door and waited. The animal jumped up to his chest in an attempt to lick his face but, thwarted by his height, finally decided to use his hand as a substitute. Ah, he thought, a grateful patient! A moment of dizziness forced him to sit down. The dog barked and pulled his shoelaces. What he needed was a little time to think, he reflected as he patted its sleek back before it settled at his feet. He looked around him. The plate on the floor, licked clean of everything but a shred of meat, meant that Tugend, the animal keeper, had already been there to feed the creature. This could be an important clue. Perhaps the fellow had removed the carcass and brought in another dog. Keats pinched his bloodshot eyes. If so, it must have been an identical twin. He picked up the dog's front paw and parted the hair. The needle mark was there.

Of one thing he was certain: Interferon, a mild viral antagonist, could by itself never have brought about this unbelievable cure. In experiments on animals it had been disappointingly ineffective. Indeed, there was no substance in medicine or surgery, or in heaven or hell, which could have overnight rescued this moribund animal from death. As an explanation there remained only the denial of reality, the conviction that the dog had never been sick, the psychotic's way. Maybe he ought to send a paper to the *American Journal of Diseases of Children* disclaiming the entire experiment. It would be called "Psychotic's Way," and the return address would be Dr. James Proust-Keats, Swann's Way, Manhattan. He took a deep breath to clear his head. The fever was obviously not doing him any good. But he was thinking clearly enough to see that the next step was to test the safety of this solution in man. That would not be so easy. Sure, sure the Salisbury group had used human subjects. But their interferon had been squirted up the nose. This time an unknown solution was going directly into the bloodstream. Where would he get volunteers for the experiment? He could try one of the prisons. If the warden asked him what he planned to inject into the convicts, he could always reply in an honest Will Rogers voice, "Damned if I know." He would probably end up in the clink himself. For this investigation there would be no long line of volunteers. Just one. He took off his jacket, rolled up his left sleeve, and walked to the refrigerator.

There were nineteen ml. in the bottle. The dose for a man, if indeed the solution was suitable for injection into man, had never been determined. Under sterile precautions he removed three ml. with a big syringe, and, covering the needle with an alcohol-soaked cottonball, laid the unit on the worktable. It suddenly occurred to him that anyone walking into the room during the next five minutes would think he was mainlining heroin. He went to the door and turned the key. Then he sat down to contemplate what he was about to do. Obviously, there was a chance that the injection would kill him. That would not be the biggest tragedy in the history of the world, he was forced to admit. Schubert had died at thirty-one, Marlowe at twenty-nine, and Alexander the Great at thirty-three. He had had his chance. God did not owe him any time. His marriage had turned his home into a disaster area. He smiled bitterly. Maybe he should have applied for Federal funds. At the hospital things were not much better. He had antagonized too many people. Although he had worked harder and longer than any man on the pediatric service, another was fated, he felt sure, to be the new director. Seniority, once the golden road to advancement, was now a barricade. Juniority was the magic carpet which flew the youngsters to the thrones of medicine over the heads of their plodding elders. Considering what the future offered, he did not have much to lose.

He stood up, straightened his left arm, swabbed the bend of his elbow with alcohol, and flexed his fingers to distend the vein. After a moment of hesitation and fear, he picked up the syringe and slipped the needle into a pale blue line under the skin of the area he had just disinfected. The fluid in front of the piston reddened at once. Very carefully he injected the three ml. into his bloodstream. The moment he pulled out the needle he knew he was not going to die. He had not felt this well in weeks. The headache and the urge to cough had disappeared. His nasal passages were clear. He could swallow without discomfort. He looked at himself in a cracked little mirror on the wall. His eyes were not bloodshot, and his nose was no longer red. He took a thermometer out of his bag and placed it under his tongue. His temperature was ninety-eight. As he replaced the instrument he noticed something peculiar about the back of his hand. He looked again. The warts, which had so irritated Annie Laurie, were gone.

This was pure charlatanism, he decided indignantly. But could a doctor practice charlatanism on himself? Impossible. Just the same, how could one conceive of a drug which would act on two conditions so totally dissimilar as a severe, febrile cold and warts? What did they have in common? Suddenly he knew. Modern scientists felt that they both were caused by viruses, warts usually by a member of the papovirus group. It was time for him to recapitulate what he had learned since yesterday. The fluid he had in the bottle destroyed the viruses which caused distemper, the common cold, and warts. Not only did it destroy the viruses, it stimulated the body cells which they had damaged to return to their normal state. He had acquired the perfect virus killer. Unfortunately, there were complications. If he treated patients with an untested drug of totally unknown composition, would not the conservative Adams medical board condemn him as a quack? Maybe they had a point. He did not feel comfortable in what he was doing. If he continued along this road, he envisioned himself ending as a barker in a county fair. He could hear himself shouting,

"Step right up, ladies and gentlemen, step right up. The miracle elixir I hold in my hand is guaranteed not to rip, rap, or wrinkle. It will stretch a mile before it tears a yard. It not only adds, subtracts, divides, and multiplies. It propagates. We have here the original Dr. Keats's Virus Killer. This reemarkable remedy is effective against any disease known to modern man and to the ancients. The Phoenicians, the Etruscans, the Hittites, and the Shit-ites all prized it above gold and precious stones. Since 1776 it has been manufactured in Kentucky caves by members of local number twelve, the famous union of villains, thieves, and scoundrels. It will cure not only tuberculosis but consumption, not only hemorrhoids but piles, not only gonorrhea but the clap. And it never hurt anybody with syphilis either. It is good for anything wrong with your anus, and not only Uranus, but Mercury, Mars, and Venus, too. It combats baldness in no time flat, or if you believe in Einstein's special theory of relativity, in no time curved. You all remember that Julius Caesar was a clean-shaven man with a head like an egg. A client of mine happily vacationing in Italy saw a bust of the great consul in the Forum Romanum. Purely as a prank, he anointed it with a single drop of the elixir. When he returned the next morning, the statue looked like Allen Ginsberg. But Keats's Virus Killer has uses of a more intimate nature. Are there not among you some men of mature years who have recently noticed a loss of potency? Ingestion of but one dose of this amazing medicine will result in the appearance of a carborundum erection whenever and as often as you wish. Please note that Carborundum is just below the diamond on Taggart's scale of hardness. To turn to the more treasured sex, are there not in this audience some shy women of still tender years who have noticed that their vaginas have become dry and rigid, doubtless due to senile atrophy? One dose of this remedy will cause the organ to become supple and moist, a veritable Garden of Eden. In a distinguished group of this size is there not one wife who has noticed a cooling of her husband's ardor? If you can persuade him to take Keats's Virus Killer regularly for one week, I promise you that he will insert his Long Branch into your Flatbush so that you can Rockaway. No offense meant, ladies, just a little family joke. By now you must imagine that this wonder-working medicine is totally beyond your reach. Do not despair. Because you are all friends of John Connally, former Secretary of the Treasury of the United States, I am prepared to offer each and every one of you an entire ml., one big thirtieth of an ounce of Keats's Virus Killer, for the unheard of, introductory bargain price of ten million dollars."

The doorknob turned. There was a violent rattling. Only then did the knocking begin. Keats turned the key and opened the door. Tugend, the animal keeper, a promoted porter, strode into the room. He was a tall man with big buttocks, a prissy, pasty Heinrich Himmler face, and a tinted pince nez. In some unknown way he had become the factotum and spy for Dr. Grant, the Director of the Laboratories. Keats disliked him for three reasons. First, he felt sure that he was an unrepentant Nazi. It had been established that he had joined the Hitler Jugend when he was fourteen and had later become a member of the Party. Nobody could figure out how he had managed to enter the United States in the early fifties. Second, he bullied everyone, the porters, cleaning women, technicians, and even the doctors. Third, he was unkind to the animals. He did nasty little things to them.

Looking around the room with as much arrogance as he could muster, and it was considerable, Tugend said, "The door was locked. Your shirtsleeve is rolled up. There is a used syringe on the table. I want to know what you were doing here. Dr. Grant would also be very much interested, I am sure, in finding out what is going on in this laboratory."

Keats turned down his shirtsleeve. He regarded the Director of Laboratories as a cold and cunning schemer. When the names of the candidates for the directorship of Pediatrics were laid before the medical board, he knew that Grant would vote against him. This Nazi lackey he held in complete contempt. He had been a young lieutenant with the outfit that had opened up Buchenwald. Twenty-eight years had not been enough to wipe out the memories of those piles of bones.

"Again I ask you," said Tugend in a shrill voice, "what were you doing here behind locked doors?"

Keats put on his jacket slowly. His football nose and massive shoulders made him look formidable. He took a quick step forward and whispered, "I was jerking off."

The animal keeper recoiled. His pasty face grew pink. "I made no such insinuation. I do not think that way. But you must admit, Doctor, that strange things are going on around here. A dog that was almost dead yesterday afternoon is now in perfect health. You yourself are cured of a severe cold in a single morning. Dr. Grant is a very inquisitive man. He likes to know everything."

"Tell him to come here alone at the stroke of midnight. We will say a Black Mass together. Then I will show him the mysteries of Murgathron, lord of the seven hells."

He walked away slowly. When he reached the door, he whirled and barked:

"Tugend!" He gave it the German pronunciation, *Too-ghent!* "Are you constipated?"

Taken aback, the animal attendant muttered, "Yes, Herr Doktor."

"This is professional advice and I want you to follow it. Take your penis in your hand. You know what your penis is, Tugend, don't you? It's that little thing that hangs down in front. Pull it until it stretches. When it is long enough, grasp it firmly and shove it up your ass. It's better than a suppository."

He walked out followed by the dog. He realized that he was becoming irritable. Well, was it surprising? He had not slept with a woman in three years. Even at his age this was not a program for attaining tranquility. He could not blame his irascibility all on Annie Laurie, though. He had always been blunt and tactless. Like the time he had unsuccessfully tried to persuade Dr. Grant to put machines in the chemistry laboratory. Now, of course, at the insistence of the medical board, it was fully automated. After the rebuff he had learned that the Director of Laboratories had written a third-rate paper largely copied from the literature on fluoridation of drinking water as a means of preventing dental caries. From that moment on he referred to him as "Caries" Grant. Since the director looked nothing like the movie actor, he was understandably miffed. Keats now admitted to himself that he had acted unwisely. If Grant had been more interested in the decay of teeth than in the decay of the laboratory, that was his business. At the time, Keats felt it would have been dishonest to keep his mouth shut. He still believed that honesty was the best policy only now he wondered whether it was not also the best means of releasing hidden aggressions. Oh well, he must abandon a self-scrutiny he was unaccustomed to and concentrate on a problem more to his liking. Would the material his friend Choate had so guilelessly given him kill other viruses? The only way to find out would be to inject it into sick children even though the stuffed shirts might throw him out of Adams for his effrontery. Along the way he might cure a few kids, even save a life. He might also ruin his career. What the hell, it would be worth it.

3

JOHN QUINCY ADAMS Hospital was founded in 1922 by Aram Gulbanian, a munitions tycoon who boasted that he was a lineal descendant of the sixth President of the United States. Since his mother's maiden name was Katchatourian, there were few who regarded his family tree as anything but a mirage. It became as real as the California redwoods the day he offered to donate twenty-five million dollars for a new hospital provided it bore his ancestor's name. A friend suggested John Adams as a substitute since it was shorter and less pretentious. Besides, he contended, John, in addition to being the second President of the United States, was John Quincy's father, a fact which would increase this genealogical triumph by one generation. But Gulbanian was stubborn. He explained that he wanted his hospital to have an impressive three-word name like Peter Bent Brigham, the illustrious Boston institution. At this his friend laughed.

"Aram, even the greatest hospitals have their ups and downs. Do you know what the interns call Peter Bent Brigham when it is going through one of its less potent phases? They refer to it as 'The Bent Peter.'"

"That will never happen to my hospital or to me either," roared the old man.

He was right as far as his own sexuality was concerned. He was seventy-two when he died after a wonderful night of love two months before the stock market crash of 1929. In the automobile on the way to the cemetery his widow turned to her bridesmaid of a half century before and said,

"It was just like our wedding night. Only he didn't hurt me the way he did then," she was careful to add.

His five-hundred-fifty-bed hospital was completed in 1922. He could never understand why a refuge for the sick could not go up as fast as a money making apartment house. In this case it did. The medical staff, all unpaid except for the full-time chiefs of X-ray and the laboratory, had to conform to a stern moral code. It was not, however, a code of sexual morality. In fact, Gulbanian had nothing against sexual immorality, a little of which he encouraged, he admitted, by refusing to allow any intern to marry during his two-year training period. Adams would be his bride, not a flesh-and-blood wife who would distract him from his profession with wiles, babies, diapering, and a thousand household stratagems. He realized that under these conditions a valve would have to be provided for the escape of the young doctors' seminal fluid, which he assumed must be under considerable pressure. To accomplish this, and, of course, for other reasons, he permitted the members of the house staff to go off duty three evenings a week. They could leave as early as six P.M. if their work was completed but they had to be back in the hospital by four the next morning. Gulbanian counted on the fact that after a few hours of illicit love they would return to the wards in the depths of the night to hold a fevered hand, calm a frightened woman, or comfort a sobbing child. And when he learned that his boys never let him down, he said that although God could see a million righteous husbands sleeping in the arms of their chaste wives whenever He chose, He would always hold these fornicating sinners closest to His heart.

Gulbanian's morality emphasized not sexual purity but work, discipline, devotion, respect, loyalty, and courage. Even then, though, there were a few avant-garde critics who called him a tyrant, the interns slaves, and his system an abomination. According to them, for the house staff to treat patients for thirty-six hours on three hours' sleep was a shameful waste of human resources. Young doctors should be in the street finding out what the community wanted, righting wrongs, fighting poverty, and crusading for civil rights. All hospital work and no sociological play made Jack Doctor a dull boy. Once after a long press conference an irate Gulbanian was asked how he would answer his opponents. He said something in Armenian and strode away. An embarrassed secretary's euphemistic translation indicated that they could all perform the act of sexual intercourse on themselves. Most people, it was clear, sided with the philanthropist. They felt that it was perfectly proper for a doctor in training to reject the joys of marriage, the responsibilities of fatherhood, the thrills of activism, and the nobility of concerned citizenship in order to treat patients for thirty-six hours on three hours' sleep.

The attending staff was a tight little paramilitary elite corps with a fixed table of organization. For instance, there were only twelve doctors each in the departments of Surgery and Medicine, five on Pediatrics. The numbers could not be increased. A new appointment could be made only if an attending died or was retired because of age, situations many of the doctors thought of as synonymous. Since four fifths of the patients were on the free wards, the attendings were rewarded not with money but with experience.

Most important of all, there were always beds available to avert an unimaginable incident in which someone who was ill would be refused admission to the hospital.

Could Gulbanian have seen Adams in 1973 he would have been amazed and probably appalled. Though the population of the United States had grown by one hundred million in fifty years, the new buildings which replaced the old did not increase the bed capacity. In contrast to ghetto hospitals, which were constantly admonished to serve the community, Adams now drew over eighty percent of its patients from outside Manhattan. The attending staff had been vastly expanded. The Department of Medicine, which once consisted of twelve physicians, now boasted of one hundred. A populous hinterland medically oriented toward the city plus over three hundred and fifty referring attendings eventually achieved the trustees' dream—total bed occupancy. Innumerable seriously ill people were refused prompt admission because Adams was full. Elective operations were planned seven weeks in advance. The administrators, the new money managers who had replaced the trustees in the day-to-day running of the hospital, were delighted. They pointed out that it was economically impractical to operate an institution with empty beds. They claimed that Adams was not full enough. And they had the statistics to prove it. Franklin D. Roosevelt once remarked that it did not help a man drowning in eight feet of water to learn that the average depth of the stream was only four feet. Similarly, it did not help a man with a bleeding stomach ulcer refused admission to the hospital because it was full to learn that the average bed occupancy was only ninety-three percent. Adams was no longer the loving mother welcoming the sick and troubled with outstretched arms. It was more like a fashionable restaurant, very hard to get into even with a reservation. The American public, which had adopted the shrug as the national gesture, shrugged and said, "Well what are you gonna do?"

The original house staff of sixteen unpaid interns had been puffed up into an army of one hundred and twenty residents who cost Adams over one and a half million dollars a year. The hospital would have run more efficiently with half as many. And each resident would have gained double the experience by seeing twice as many patients and working harder. In fact the medical board had difficulty each year filling all the unnecessary positions it had itself created. It was forced to bring in foreign graduates. But it felt it must persist in its recruiting efforts in order to preserve Adams's prestige. Just as an African chief's social standing was determined by the size of his herds and a sultan's by the size of his harem, so a hospital's importance was in part determined by the number of residents it could display. It was argued that the leading institutions were obligated to provide such a large number of residencies in order to train doctors for an America sadly in need of them. Unfortunately the young men whom Adams educated did not go to Watts, Harlem, or Appalachia. They either returned to their homelands or opened offices in the affluent suburbs.

There was one change in John Quincy Adams that Gulbanian would have understood and perhaps even endorsed. By 1967 the trustees could no longer ignore the fact that it was becoming increasingly difficult to persuade the seven unpaid directors who made up the medical board to steal enough time from their private practices to run their departments and fulfill their committee assignments. To remedy this situation they decided to give each director a salary of thirty-five thousand dollars a year to do his job efficiently instead of perfunctorily. The positions at once became much more desirable since to the power and prestige they had all along conferred was now added a handsome income. The recipients of this generosity were allowed to pursue the private practice of medicine just as they had before.

They responded promptly to the crack of the financial whip; all except Evan Dummer, the head of Pediatrics. In his case the trustees were flogging a dray horse at Epsom Downs. By 1970 his department had dwindled to forty beds, at least one third of which were usually unoccupied. Of the few children who were treated on the seventh floor, half belonged to surgery and the surgical specialties. To the businessmen and corporation lawyers on the governing board empty beds were an indication of inefficiency and failure. To be merciful to the head of a department which had a low census was a sign of softness. Besides, in a world where residents were a director's currency, Dummer was a poor man. He had only two. Prodded by Hexter, the administrator, the trustees were on the verge of asking Dummer to resign at once instead of allowing him to stay on for three more years, when he would automatically leave with honor at the mandatory retirement age of sixty-five.

He was not to blame for the empty beds in the pediatric division, a regrettable condition, at least from the hospital's point of view, caused by the migration to the suburbs and the diminution of significant illness in the young. But he was a poor chief. A handsome man, he lacked the brains to match his powerful features. At the medical board meetings he spoke frequently but without authority. To his fellow directors he was a nag; to his subordinates a castrative milquetoast. Keats called him the Catabolic Kid. It was an accurate designation. He managed to take part in the destruction of any enterprise with which he was connected.

He decided to seek the help of Dr. Thomas Locke, Professor of Pediatrics at the Medical Center. The illustrious pediatrician's office there was noted as much for its beautiful simplicity as for a total absence of toys, balloons, and lollipops. He was a research man and an executive, not a clinician. After listening to Dummer's description of the situation at Adams, Locke expressed surprise that he had been chosen as the recipient of such confidential information.

"It's quite simple," replied Dummer. "I came here to ask you for one of your bright young men. Perhaps he could help me turn things around."

Locke thought for a moment and said, "I'm interested in the university, the Medical Center, and my own department. I don't like to send young men to pluck other people's chestnuts from the fire. However, when I do, I also supply enough residents to put the ailing department on its feet. Every year I must turn down at least forty applicants for my residencies. In certain situations I suggest that some of them go to a hospital of my choice. They usually do."

"I'm not surprised."

"I'm wondering what we at the Medical Center would get out of this arrangement. This might be something. You will reach the mandatory retirement age in three years, I believe. If I breathe life into your department, I would want my man to get your job when you leave."

Dummer did not protest.

For the sake of decency Locke held his hand forward. "I know, I know. He doesn't deserve it and you have men who do. But we are not talking about what he deserves. We are talking about what he is going to get. If he eventually does become director, you need have no fear. The university and the Medical Center would not demand control of your department." He flashed a charming smile. "All we would ask for is to have something to say. Are we in agreement?"

"In perfect agreement."

"You don't have to discuss all the ramifications of our little chat with your medical board at this time. Everything will fall into place eventually."

"May I ask whom you have in mind?"

Locke shrugged. "I've been thinking of Tunbridge Wells, but I don't know whether he would take the job."

"That boy already has one of the biggest practices in New York. I can't figure out how he does it."

Locke grinned sardonically. "Ability, pure ability."

Then he stood up, ushered Dummer to the door, and dismissed him with a handshake. Before he sat down at his desk he dialed the page operator.

Tunbridge Wells was the only son of a well-to-do and socially prominent Westchester family. When he was twenty-one, his maternal grandmother died, leaving him three hundred thousand dollars in gilt-edged securities. After graduating from Yale Medical School, he worked diligently for four years on Dr. Locke's house staff, serving as chief resident at the end. His specialty, an innocent heart murmur, and a letter from his chief, protected him from the draft. As soon as he entered private practice he was given a minor position in the pediatric division, which obliged him to work a half afternoon a week in the outpatient clinic, attend the Wednesday morning conference, and help occasionally with the training of the residents. The unimportance of his duties did not disturb him. Advancement in the academic world was not his ambition. He had only one goal —to make money. It was indeed strange that he had chosen the practice of pediatrics in Manhattan to attain it. It was as if a young man who was determined to spend his life seducing women decided to further his aim by entering a monastery. Considering his choice of a specialty, Wells's financial success was phenomenal. By the time he was thirty-five he was making seventy thousand dollars a year. If he had gone into general surgery, his friends said, he would be earning a quarter of a million. But he was not good with his hands. He had no mechanical ability. And, as he so frankly admitted, he did not like the idea of treating smelly old men and women.

He was neither a very good pediatrician nor a very bad one. He had never written a paper for a medical periodical. He read little of the scientific literature. But he was a superb salesman. It was this ability which made patients flock to his office. Inordinately handsome, tall and lean with a Byronesque air, he caused a greater rise in the mothers' pulse rates by his looks than a fall in their children's temperatures by his use of antibiotics. Optimistic and expansive, he managed to create the impression that he knew everyone of consequence, that he was a ticket fixer, an intimate of influential politicians, a man who could get things done. If a friend complained that Yale had turned down his son, he would reply, "You should have spoken to me. I went to college with the dean's nephew." If another confessed that his boy was out of work, he would reassure him with, "I'll take care of it. Put it from your mind. Is U. S. Steel good enough for him? I treat the children of the executive vice-president." His failure to report on any progress with U. S. Steel later on would be overlooked when the boy found a job on his own. No one held Wells's bluffing against him, though. After all, he peddled hope.

Twice a year he gave a deck-sweeping cocktail party at the Waldorf to even the score with all the people who had invited him to dinner. The affairs were so obviously tax deductible that the Internal Revenue Service never quibbled. Guests were frequently heard to say that he had the busiest and most fashionable pediatric practice in town. They were not far from the mark.

Quite early in his career he decided not to marry. To his patients he said, "I see too many wonderful children in my office to feel the need for more." He had coitus frequently; affairs never. He chose married women as his bed partners first because they would almost certainly be on the pill, second because they were probably more knowledgeable, and third because there was less danger of entanglement. His system was so effective that he often wished he could patent it. Without saying a word he was able to convey the fact that going to bed with him was a once-in-a-lifetime occurrence, like a trip to

Hong Kong, kissing the Blarney Stone, or visiting the Kremlin. True, if the woman did not attempt to ensnare him, an encore was a distinct possibility. His genius lay in his ability to make a previously faithful wife believe that it was she who had arranged the roll in the hay to relieve her tensions. His self-conferred description, steel-prick Wells, was deserved. He was polite and pleasant afterward. No woman who had spent an hour with him ever felt guilty the next day.

He answered the page on the first ring, and was in Dr. Locke's office in three minutes.

"Bridge," said the eminent pediatrician, "I've just had a visit with Evan Dummer. If the first 'e' is pronounced like the two in 'eel,' no man was ever more appropriately named. Evidently his department is in bad shape. The trustees at Adams are thinking of dumping him. He wants me to let him have one of my bright young men to help him hold his job for three more years." He smiled. "Now you know that you aren't one of my bright young men. You never could be. By a happy coincidence, though, a bright young man is not what the people at Adams need. He would only arouse their suspicion. What they need is a shrewd young man who gets along."

"What would my duties be, sir?"

"To keep Dummer in the good graces of the medical board and the trustees for three years."

"And then?"

"To take his job."

Wells seemed dumbfounded. "But they must have some senior men there waiting for the promotion. Dr. Keats in particular is pretty good, isn't he?"

"Outstanding. One of the best clinicians in town. And he's written some good papers, too, on Rh, exchange transfusions, blood iron, and rheumatic heart disease. He's the logical man for the job. But he doesn't have a chance. I wouldn't send you there if he did. He's too blunt, too abrasive, maybe even too honest." He paused. "And too old. In 1973 you will be thirty-eight. You will have attained just the right degree of *immaturity* for the job. Keats has solid achievement behind him. You've never written an article. But achievement is no longer important in choosing a chief. Today the magic word, the open sesame, is *promise*. Promise is the great carrot young doctors dangle before the snouts of hospitals." He sighed. "You may wonder why medical boards and trustees react this way. Well, achievement is the meal they had last week. Promise is the banquet they've been invited to tonight."

"Wasn't Keats a great football player long ago?"

"Oh, I wouldn't say he was great. He had no finesse, no moves. His repertoire consisted of bulling his way through the middle of the line for four yards." He smiled. "But you could always count on him for four yards."

"Did you ever play opposite him?"

"Once a year at tackle for Princeton. He always seemed to go through my side of the line."

"I don't mean to change the subject, sir, but is there any salary involved?"

"I'm surprised that you ask." He gave a mocking smile. "I thought you were idealistic, like the barefoot doctors of China. Yes, there is a salary. Adams now pays its directors thirty-five thousand dollars a year for the part-time service they used to give for nothing."

"Very nice. Thank you for throwing this opportunity my way."

"Let me tell you about the hierarchy at Adams. In ascending order of power it is assistant adjunct, adjunct, associate, attending, and director. Everyone goes in as an assistant adjunct. I want you, however, to insist on going in as an associate. Whenever anyone offers you a position you can afford to turn down, always make demands. Keats is a full attending. You'll jump over his head in three years." He looked hard at Wells. "The first thing you should do when they make you an associate is to set up a paper service for Dummer. You know how to do that, don't you?"

"Certainly. I was your chief resident."

"Next, convince Dummer that only the director and the residents count. Persuade him to make rounds with the residents alone. Get him to banish the members of the attending staff from all rounds, even grand rounds. In that way he won't have any rivals, and you won't either. Most of the older men know more than he does. The idea is to push them to the side."

"That's a heady cocktail, sir, wisdom with a dash of cunning."

"Thank you for the bartender's compliment." He smiled thinly. "I hear you go to bed with the mothers of your little patients."

"Oh, no, sir. Only with some of them."

Locke nodded approvingly. "I've taught you that a man should never overestimate his laboratory accomplishments. I see that you have extended this maxim to the bedroom. Do you find that your sexual prowess helps you in your practice?"

"I don't think so. It's something that's just thrown in occasionally, like a door prize."

"Another cocktail. Realism with a dash of modesty. You know, Bridge, Dr. Keats has a beautiful young wife. If I were you I wouldn't make her my first conquest."

"Your warning is academic. I'm sure she wouldn't have anything to do with me."

"I'm not so sure. I hear you are a second Paris, the Greek as well as the city."

"I never take a woman away from her husband. Prisoners of love like prisoners of war have to be fed."

"A sensible reason is often more compelling than a moral one." Locke stroked his chin. "I dislike leaving so delicious a discussion, but we must go on to something more important. You will, of course, let me know what goes on at Adams. I cannot send battalions of residents to an unknown land. To underline my point I might add that if you become director and prove cooperative, I might arrange for a loose affiliation between the Department of Pediatrics at Adams and the medical school here."

"Dr. Locke, you will continue to be my chief for the next ten years as you have been for the last."

Locke laughed scornfully. "Don't be offended, Bridge, but I think Adams is going to get exactly what it deserves."

On May first, 1970, Tunbridge Wells was appointed Associate Pediatrician to John Quincy Adams Hospital. On July first twelve residents began their training in the Department of Pediatrics. The medical board and the trustees were quick to see the connection. In September the schedule appeared. The front page was filled with four long columns labeled first, second, third, and fourth on call, each containing the name of a pediatric resident for every day of the month. First-on-call slept in the hospital. The other three left at five in the afternoon to hurry home to their families. No one ever bothered to find out if they were really available. Thus of the twelve residents, one or at most two spent the night on duty at Adams. If the word *resident* means "one who resides permanently in a place," no group was ever more grossly misnamed. Page two had the roster of those who were assigned to the nursery, the clinics, the emergency room, and the seventh floor itself. On the third page the attendings and their tasks were listed. Each was to make rounds once a month instead of four times a week, and never with Dr. Dummer. Each was to lecture to the residents once a month. There were no other duties. Wells was proud of his creation. He had given his chief a beautiful paper service and at the same time effectively if not officially removed competitors from the pediatric arena. He saw to it that the monthly schedules were posted all over the hospital and sent them regularly to the members of the medical board, the administrators, and the nursing office. Twice he mailed a copy to the chairman of the board of trustees—by mistake. The plan to dump Dummer was abruptly dropped.

The following year there were fourteen residents. Since the average medical-pediatric census was only thirteen, there were often more residents than patients. Although Wells sent many of his private patients into the hospital, including some who were not sick enough to deserve admission, the number of unoccupied beds did not significantly diminish. At this point he obtained his chief's consent to carry out what became known as operation on-duty-elsewhere. He arranged for the residents to go to any children's hospital of their choice in England or Europe for three months. Foreign countries were glad to get American currency. Next, he persuaded Dr. Locke to allow them to spend a three-month observation period at the Medical Center. Strengthened by these accomplishments, he found it easy to obtain similar courtesies from other hospitals in New York State. Finally, he induced a few of his wealthy patients to set up a fund so that the members of the house staff could go to medical conventions anywhere in the United States. There were times when it seemed as if there were more residents on-duty-elsewhere than in the hospital itself. Their password became "Join Adams and See the World." And they were delighted, especially since they continued to be paid while they roamed. Of course, they did not do much work for the Department of Pediatrics, but then there was not much work to be done. Wells became something of a patron saint of the young.

He was popular with the attendings as well—with all, that is, except those of his own department. His large practice enabled him to send lucrative cases to the directors of the various specialty departments. After all, it was they who had the votes. But he sent many patients to doctors in the lower echelons as well. You never knew who could do you a favor. He added another deck sweeper at the Waldorf, this one for doctors, head nurses, administrators, key personnel, and even a few trustees at Adams. For the obstetricians who referred patients to him he held little dinner parties at Twenty One, Grenouille, and Lutece. The wives were always invited. He did not have a family to support and the entertainment was income-tax deductible. By 1973 he was regarded as a coming man.

In fact at the Adams alumni dinner dance held early in October at the Hotel Hilton people were openly prophesying that he would be the next director of Pediatrics. He had been placed next to Dummer at the table reserved for pediatricians. Keats whispered in Annie Laurie's ear, "Wells is sitting at the right hand of the chief like the Son of God." Mrs. Dummer, who was sixty-three, gave him motherly glances. Those of the other wives were far less maternal.

After dinner Dummer took him by the elbow and guided him to a corner of the ballroom for another of the father-to-son chats he enjoyed giving. Adams was dancing to the tunes of the twenties. Keats and Annie Laurie were seated nearby, looking away from each other. She did not dance with him because she thought him clumsy. Besides, he was sniffling and coughing. Wells and Dummer found themselves staring at her.

"Beautiful but cold, isn't she?" said the director.

"I wonder whether there's a fire in the igloo," said his companion.

"Why don't you ask her to dance?"

Wells walked across the floor and after a "May I?" to Keats, held out his hand to her. The band was playing Gershwin's "Embraceable You." The tempo was slow, the timbre stirring. After dancing for several minutes she looked up at him and asked,

"Do you snore?"

"Not since I had my tonsils and adenoids removed. I was six at the time."

No other words passed between them.

As soon as he returned, Dummer asked, "Does she dance well?"

"I don't know but she's built like a brick shit house."

Where women were concerned, Dummer enjoyed being treated like one of the boys. He smiled and put his arm around the younger man's shoulders. "You'd better not let her husband hear you say that."

"I'm sure he knows it," said Wells. Then he laughed and added, "If I can't seduce that woman and with your help beat her husband out of the directorship, I'll leave town. I simply can't give up this once-in-a-lifetime chance of screwing a husband and wife."

Dummer was shocked, but he felt a strange excitement. He decided that Wells was joking.

THE FRIDAY after Keats had injected the virus killer into his bloodstream, he received a telephone call from Mrs. Rush.

"Nancy has had one hundred and two and spots on her body for two days. It looks like chickenpox."

Keats waited, but she said nothing more. "Bring her to the office at three," he said. "I won't be seeing patients then." Mrs. Rush's silence continued. "Or if you wish," he said, "I'll make a house call."

"We're going to Easthampton for the weekend in a few minutes. My husband is loading the car."

"I wouldn't recommend a three-hour automobile trip for a child with a temperature of one hundred and two."

"I know it must sound strange," she said, "but we simply have to go. It's just one of those things. And we have to take Nancy because the maids have the weekend off." There was a long pause. "Her school is full of chickenpox. I thought perhaps you could prescribe something over the phone."

"I can't prescribe anything until I see her."

The Rushes were one of many couples who having bought costly houses in Easthampton were determined to get a return on their investment. During weekends and school holidays in autumn, winter, and spring, the children, often suffering from colds, coughs, and fevers, were driven there regardless of the weather so that the parents could observe the maxim "Waste not, want not." In the summer when the weather was mild and beautiful, the children did not go to Easthampton. They went to camp.

At noon on Saturday Mrs. Rush called him again, this time from Easthampton. "She's terribly sick now. And it all happened so suddenly. The pediatrician here thinks she has pneumonia in addition to chickenpox. And something called disseminated intravascular coagulation. There are big, bloody places all over her body."

Again there was a long silence. She was one of those people, he decided, who did not believe in asking a doctor for help. She had stated the facts. She had done her duty. The rest was up to him.

"What would you like me to do?" he asked.

"Do you think she can stand the trip back to New York?"

"I can't tell from here. But in case you need me, I'll be available all afternoon and all night."

At three in the afternoon she telephoned that they were home. He drove there in four minutes, putting a prescription blank with the Rushes' Park Avenue address and apartment number under the windshield wiper of his double-parked car. When the elevator came down at last, it was filled with luggage and laughing passengers who did not seem to be in a hurry to get out. The moment it emptied he growled the patient's name at the operator, who, seeing the expression on the doctor's face, took the car up at once without waiting for the people who were at that moment entering the lobby.

Mr. and Mrs. Rush were standing in the doorway. After greeting them, Keats walked to the toilet to wash his hands. Then he entered the bedroom quietly. A glance at Nancy convinced him that the prognosis was grave. She was lying on her back in bed, slipping into unconsciousness. Even before he took his stethoscope out of his bag, he could tell from the rapid breathing, the grunting expirations, and the flaring of the nostrils that she had pneumonia. Undressing the seven-year-old girl was a formidable undertaking. Her buttonless slip-on pajama top could not be so easily slipped off. The manufacturers had achieved this one-way triumph by making the neck opening three sizes too small. Freeing her reminded him of extracting a newborn from its mother in a difficult breach delivery, the kind in which the baby's buttocks come out first. With Mrs. Rush holding the inverted pajama top firmly over Nancy's head, he managed to pull her through at last. Not only her scalp and face but her torso and extremities were covered with chickenpox blisters. But these were no ordinary blisters. Each was filled with blood. And everywhere under the skin were spreading hemorrhages. Inside the mouth, which he examined with a pen light and a tongue blade, there were clusters of ulcers. He pulled down both lower lids. The right eye was violently inflamed because of a pock resting directly on the cornea. Mrs. Rush had joined her husband at the other end of the room. "I had a premonition we should never have gone to Easthampton," she whispered to him. "We should never have bought the house. If anything happens to Nancy, I'm going to make you sell it."

"All right, all right!" said her husband. "We made an error in judgment. Millions of kids get chickenpox. How many end up like our poor little girl? How could we have guessed what would happen?"

"It's that damn tennis of yours. You would think Easthampton was Wimbledon."

"Since when is exercise a sin? You need it, too. That's why I like to see you play golf."

Mrs. Rush looked at Nancy and started to cry. "To hell with golf. I'll never break a hundred after this." She wiped her eyes. "We're being punished. But I can't understand why God would want to take it out on a little girl."

"Maybe the doctor will make her better," said Mr. Rush.

"Suppose he doesn't," said his wife.

Keats looked at them. "Do you mind being quiet for a moment? I'm going to examine her lungs."

He turned Nancy on her chest and listened to her back with his stethoscope. He was not surprised to hear crepitant rales, those tiny crackles which are typical of pneumonia. After he had completed the examination he walked into the living room with Mrs. Rush. Her husband patted Nancy's foot and followed them. As soon as they sat down, Keats said,

"She has a rare hemorrhagic form of chickenpox and chickenpox pneumonia. She's very sick."

"Is there any hope?" asked Mr. Rush.

"Miracles can happen."

"What's the matter with her eye, Doctor?"

"There's a pock directly on her cornea."

"Can anything be done about it?"

Keats shrugged. "If she should survive, a corneal transplant, perhaps." He rose. "I'm going to try to get something for her, some varicella-zoster immune globulin. It often prevents chickenpox after the child has been exposed. Maybe it will have a favorable effect after the disease has taken hold. May I use your phone?" Rush ushered him into the master bedroom and closed the door.

Seated on the double bed with his hand on the telephone, Keats knew that there were times when it was impossible to get this biological product. It had never really been commercially available. Yet he remembered that his pharmacy, now the largest supplier of vaccines, sera, and drugs in the city, had more than once obtained unusual biologicals for him when the quest seemed hopeless. Unfortunately, the store closed at six o'clock on Friday evenings and did not open until nine on Monday morning. He looked at his watch. It was three forty-five. Someone might be in the store this Saturday afternoon taking inventory or working on the books. He waited for the telephone to buzz ten times before he hung up. He thought of using cortisone and heparin, but realized at once that they would probably be ineffective and dangerous. Blood-coagulation studies would be informative, but he had so little time. Then he remembered that he had recently read in the *New York State Medical Journal* that varicella-zoster immune globulin could be obtained from Dr. Thomas Locke at the Medical Center. He looked at his watch again. No full-time professor of pediatrics would be sitting in his office at ten minutes to four on a beautiful Saturday afternoon in October. True, quite true, but Keats felt certain that he knew where he could be found. He would be sitting in front of the television set in his living room in Larchmont watching the Princeton game which was being played this week in Athens, Georgia. He felt equally certain that his former football opponent would not willingly answer the telephone. If forced to by the threat of an emergency, he would hardly be in the mood to give away a large amount of a drug in such short supply as varicella-zoster immune globulin. Keats realized that he would simply have to wait until the game was over.

As soon as he entered the living room he saw that he had interrupted a quarrel between the Rushes. Mr. Rush stood up.

"Did you get what you wanted for Nancy?"

"Not yet," answered Keats.

He went to the television set and, after a murmured, "May I?" turned on the Princeton-Georgia game. The camera, focused on the scoreboard, indicated that Princeton was ahead fourteen to ten in the fourth quarter. There were six minutes still to play. He left the set turned on and walked into Nancy's bedroom. It would have been cruel, he felt, to tell the Rushes about the work habits of medical-school professors, or to mention that Tom Locke, the guardian of the drug he thought their daughter needed, had been Princeton's star tackle thirty-five years before. Let them regard their pediatrician as an eccentric if they wished.

Nancy was lying in bed with her eyes closed in the same position as before. The maid, who had been hastily recalled because of the emergency, was standing in the corner. She shook her head sadly. After a moment's hesitation, he bent down and with his lips an inch from the child's ear called out her name. There was no response. The poor thing was stuporous. He pulled a chair to the side of the bed and sat down with his chin resting in the palm of his hand. The position reminded him of Sir Luke Fildes's most famous painting, "Doctor," a great favorite of his father's and of Victorian England's. A reproduction hung in the office in the old brownstone house on East 65th Street where he had spent most of his childhood. When his father was out making house calls, he would often stand in front of the picture for minutes at a time dreaming that some day he would be that kind of a doctor. Fildes's work depicts a miserably furnished hovel with the grieving parents standing inconspicuously in the background darkness. Bathed in light in front are the doctor and the patient. The critically ill little girl lies across two pillow-covered chairs. Evidently her father cannot afford to buy her a bed. The doctor, dressed in a beautifully cut frock coat, high collar and silk tie, is seated beside her, his bearded chin resting in his upturned palm. On his face there is an expression of sadness and compassion. Anyone can see he is not going to send a bill. When Keats grew up, he came to believe that the doctor in the picture was not so much saddened as puzzled. He was trying to figure out what to do. Well, what *could* he do? What could any doctor have done with that Victorian pharmacopeia of useless drugs? Although Keats was in a Park Avenue apartment instead of a hovel with all the resources of modern medicine at his command, he felt as frustrated as Fildes's doctor who sat by a sick child in a long dead England. Keats could not even admit her to Adams. The hospital did not accept patients with contagious diseases.

After a few minutes he walked into the living room and stood in front of the television set. The score was still fourteen to ten in favor of Princeton but with four minutes left to play. The Georgia quarterback faded into the pocket and threw a long pass, which a Princeton safety man easily batted down. Jesus, said Keats to himself, an incomplete pass stops the clock. The longer this goddamn game takes the worse it is for Nancy.

"Whom are you rooting for, Doctor?" asked Rush.

"Princeton," said Keats. Without another word he walked to his patient's room.

"There's something wrong with that man," said Mrs. Rush. "He's mad. My little girl is dying, and he comes popping in here every minute to look at the score."

"Stop it!" said her husband. "He's under a strain, too."

"Oh, you're as bad as he is. I saw you looking at the television set out of the corner of your eye. What is he, some kind of a football nut?"

"He was a great fullback in the old days."

"He looks it with those huge shoulders and that bent football nose. Don't tell me a thug like that played for Princeton?"

"No, no, for Columbia. My father says he saw him rip the Princeton line to shreds one afternoon thirty-five years ago."

"Then why does he root for Princeton?"

Her husband shrugged.

She nudged him as footsteps sounded in the corridor. "Here he comes to find out what the score is."

Keats walked up to the television set just as she had predicted. The score was fourteen–ten, Princeton leading with one minute left to go. Unfortunately, it was second down and Georgia had the ball on Princeton's four-yard line. If they rammed over the touchdown, Keats was convinced that Locke would be a hard man to deal with. Georgia tried a quarterback sneak. Beautiful, said Keats to himself, they're running the wrong play. He was right. It didn't gain an inch. A reverse on third down was equally unsuccessful. For the last down they would have to give the ball to the fullback, he knew, just as they should have done all along. The quarterback spun and handed the ball to number fourteen. Wonderful, wonderful shouted Keats to himself, the slow, stupid bastard is trying an end run. The Princeton middle linebacker came up fast and threw him for a three-yard loss. The whistle blew. The gun sounded. The game was over. Smiling grimly, Keats turned off the set, walked into the master bedroom, and closed the door.

Locke answered the telephone on the first ring. He was evidently expecting calls from old Princetonians.

After identifying himself, Keats said, "You had some tough boys in there today. Congratulations."

"We were lucky. Georgia didn't have a Jim Keats in the backfield."

You're damned right, said Keats to himself. I could carry five ounces of ball and thirty pounds of extra fat into the Princeton end zone any day. But out loud all he said was,

"Thanks. You're trying to make up for the times you smeared me on the line of scrimmage."

"It wasn't often."

"I took the liberty of calling you to discuss the case of a seven-year-old girl who has hemorrhagic varicella, probably disseminated intravascular coagulation, a lesion on the right cornea, and varicella pneumonia. Her temperature is one hundred and five, and she is comatose." He gave a detailed description of the clinical picture. Then he paused. "I wonder whether you could let me have some varicella-zoster immune globulin."

"I don't have any," answered Locke. "We have a large number of children with leukemia on the pediatric service, all under cortisone therapy. One of them got chickenpox and died. As you can imagine, it became necessary to protect the others. A leukemic child who contracts varicella while on steroids is in mortal peril. We gave immune globulin on a large scale. Not a child came down with chickenpox, I'm happy to say. But we used up all our immune globulin in the process. I'm afraid the current epidemic has put the other medical centers in the same boat."

"Do you think I could get some from the National Institutes of Health?"

"Even if they had it, they wouldn't fly it up until Monday. Your little girl will be dead by then."

"I'm sure of it."

"A favorite patient, of course."

"Of course."

"Let me tell you something. It won't help her, but it may help you. It certainly makes things easier for me. No amount of immune globulin could save that child."

Keats thanked him and hung up. He stared at the floor for a little while. Then he raised his head. From the moment he had first examined Nancy he had been struggling, perhaps without knowing it, with the urge to use the virus killer. It was all very well for him to have blustered to himself that he was going to test its effectiveness by injecting it into children. Now he must make a decision that would affect a flesh-and-blood girl, not a research project. True, he had introduced it into his own vein with only the most beneficial results. But he weighed two hundred and forty pounds, the patient fifty-one. Suppose a child's body was too weak and immature to withstand this mysteriously potent medication? Suppose Nancy gasped and died before he could withdraw the needle? Well, she was going to die anyway. Her imminent death would not absolve him, however. A man who killed a dying child was nonetheless a murderer.

He decided to go to a quiet place where he could resolve his dilemma undisturbed. In his little laboratory at Adams, close to the cause of his predicament, he would come to a decision. He walked into the living room and said to the Rushes, "I can't get any immune globulin for Nancy. I'm going to try to get something else."

When he reached the street he saw that there was a twenty-five-dollar ticket on his windshield. He felt the same kind of rage that used to possess him when some huge tackle chopped him as he hit the line for Columbia. For the past thirty years he had given fifty percent of his time and fifty percent of his strength to treating indigent children of the City of New York free of charge. For this he did not expect a ticker-tape parade, a scroll, or even a pat on the back. All he wanted was freedom from harassment. Although a long and detailed letter of explanation to the New York County Medical Society might result in a revocation of the fine, it could not abolish his present irritation. What disturbed him most was the fact that his anger took his mind off his work and prevented him from having a clear head when he needed one most. He got into his car and drove to Adams. As usual, there were no parking places. He double parked, flipping down the visor with his location in the hospital attached to it. He left the ticket on the windshield hoping that the tax collectors in blue would be fooled by the ruse.

He saw Tugend out of the corner of his eye as soon as he entered the research building. Closing the door of his laboratory, he took off his jacket and carried the interferon solution from the icebox to the worktable. After he had been seated for a minute, he realized that he had his arm around the virus killer as if it were the head of a sleeping bride. There was a gentle knock on the door. He stood up. If that Nazi bastard walked in, he said to himself, he was going to let him have one of those perfect blocks he used to hit Tom Locke with in the old days. The soft tapping was repeated. Keats sighed and opened the door. The animal keeper entered slowly and let his little spy's eyes roam over the room. They finally darted to the pediatrician's shirtsleeves to determine whether they had just been turned down. Grant's informer, thought Keats, was panning for mud in the great Adams muck-rush.

"I came to see if I could help," said Tugend. "Is there anything I can do?"

"Yeh," answered Keats. "Fuck off."

He was surprised to see such a flabby man move so quickly. They ought to make him an honorary traffic cop with the privilege of ticketing only doctors' cars.

He walked to the worktable. There was a scratching at the door. As soon as he opened it, the dog trotted in. He pointed his finger at the animal and said, "I saved your life. Now let me try to save a little girl." The dog lay down and began to lick its paws. This place was getting to be busier than Grand Central Station, he decided. He sat down at last to think.

The Food and Drug Administration had not, of course, released the virus killer for general use. It would first have to be tested on many animals, and then, in the hands of chosen full-time investigators, on adults and children. The quantity of drug needed would be enormous, the process time consuming. Nevertheless, any doctor who injected a patient with a drug not yet approved by the FDA did so at his peril. If Keats administered the virus killer to Nancy and she died, Mrs. Rush would probably sue him even though he was not responsible for the death. Since he had used an unauthorized drug, his malpractice insurance company might not pay the out-of-court settlement that would be the best he could hope for. Suits against physicians no longer had to have merit, only nuisance value. He shook his head. This line of reasoning was bringing him no closer to a decision. Only two questions had to be answered. One, would Nancy die if he withheld the virus killer? The answer was assuredly yes. Two, was there a chance, however small, that she might live if he gave it to her? Again the answer was yes. He reached into a drawer and brought out a sterile pipette. The dose for children had not been determined. He transferred two ml. from the bottle to a glass tube.

On the way to the Rushes' he decided not to discuss with them the origin and nature of the solution he was about to inject into their daughter. How could he justify to these people the administration of a medication whose composition was unknown? The somber maid ushered him into Nancy's room, now darkened by the turned down Venetian blinds except in the region of the bed, which was brightly illuminated by a floor lamp. At first he did not see the parents standing motionless against the far wall. As soon as he nodded to them, he sat down in the chair next to the bed feeling again like the doctor in Fildes's picture. Not quite, though. The hovel had been replaced by a luxurious apartment, and the vast arsenal of useless Victorian drugs by the virus killer. Nancy was unconscious. Her breathing was labored. With difficulty he was able to pull her tight-fitting pajama sleeve above her elbow. He turned her hand palm upward on the bed and told the maid to hold her wrist. Next he unwrapped a sterile, five-ml. disposable syringe he kept in his bag, and with it removed the solution from the glass tube. As soon as he applied the tourniquet to Nancy's arm, he slipped the needle into the small vein at the bend of the elbow with practiced ease. Almost in one motion he flipped off the tourniquet and injected the virus killer directly into her bloodstream. The needle was out and he was pressing an alcohol-soaked cottonball on the tiny break in the skin before the maid realized what had happened. When he was satisfied that there would be no bleeding, he pulled down the sleeve. For the next half hour he watched the patient with frenzied intensity. There was no change. He sat there another half hour. She looked exactly as she had before the injection. Well, what did he expect, nightingales and larks and sweet, scented meadows, the laying on of the hands and the king's touch? Or a glimpse of Orpheus in the doorway playing his lute so beguilingly that Nancy would turn away from her journey into the land of the dead? Come to think of it, Orpheus hadn't done so well by his girl, either. Everybody, everything, had limitations. The virus killer, too. He pulled up Nancy's pajama top so that he could see her chest and abdomen. The hemorrhagic rash was appalling. But the respiratory rate seemed slower. He timed it. It was twenty-five to the minute, almost normal for her age. And her skin was cool. He pulled down her pajama top and looked at her face. She opened her good eye.

He stood up and said, "I'll be back at seven."

As soon as Mrs. Rush heard the front door close, she said to her husband, "There's something strange about that man."

"A man has to be strange to be a pediatrician," he answered, "with all that crying and the low fees."

Keats drove to Adams with the ticket on his windshield like an amulet to ward off evil. He was worried about the Prince boy, a patient on the seventh floor who had been having unexplained fever for five days. Another thorough physical examination revealed nothing abnormal. Seated next to the bed, Keats read through the chart carefully. The X-ray and laboratory reports were run-of-the-mill. By exclusion, he reasoned, the boy must have a viral infection. He smiled. When he was young, he had made many house calls in elevatorless tenements. Most of his patients managed to live on the top floor. It did not seem to matter whether the child's presenting symptom was cough, pain in the chest, vomiting, headache, dizziness, or sore throat. The mother's diagnosis, delivered in perfect dactylic trimeter, was always, "It MUSTa bin SUMPin he ET." Medicine had made great strides since then, he said to himself. The mother's diagnosis had been replaced by the doctor's, which, though still couched in dactylic trimeter, ran, "It LOOKS like a VIrus to ME." The new nomenclature was so much more impressive than the old. As he picked up his bag before returning to Nancy, he glanced at his patient. He seemed unusually quiet for an eleven-year-old boy.

Mr. Rush, smiling broadly, opened the door for the doctor seconds after the bell rang. Mrs. Rush seemed less tense but there was a wary glint in her eye. The three walked to Nancy's bedroom. She was sitting on the floor playing with her dolls.

"Get into bed," Keats ordered sternly.

She obeyed at once and lay meekly on her back. He tried to lift her buttonless pajama top over her head, but the manufacturer had cunningly designed it so that although it could be put on without any trouble, it could not be so easily pulled off. He drew it down to her waist and slit it open from top to bottom with the bandage scissors he had removed from his bag. He had saved her life, he reasoned, he was entitled to ruin her pajamas. The rash had completely disappeared. Her skin had never been more beautiful. He pulled down both lower lids. Her eyes were normal, the irises that crystalline, transparent blue seen only in children. She was breathing easily. Although he listened to her chest with his stethoscope for over a minute, he could not hear a single rale. Her throat was clear. Her temperature, ninety-eight. The rest of the physical examination was unremarkable. He put his instruments in his bag and stood up.

Nancy stood up too. "Can I go to school tomorrow?"

"No."

"Why?"

"Because it's Sunday."

She laughed. "Silly! Can I go Monday?"

"The Health Department says you have to stay home until Thursday."

She walked by his side through the corridor, followed by her parents.

"When I grow up I'm going to be a doctor," she said.

"I have a better idea," said Keats. "Marry a doctor."

She shook her head. When they reached the foyer, she said,

"If you were nine, I would marry you, though."

He found her remark quite sensible. At seven, her age, he would have been too immature. Obviously, nine was just right for a successful marriage. Bowing gravely from the waist, he said,

"In the name of the nine-year-old boy I once was, I accept."

"Nancy," her mother said sharply, "go back to your room and put on your bathrobe. And close the door."

As soon as she heard the click, she turned to Keats and said, "I think you owe us an explanation."

"For what?"

"For everything. Nancy was dying. Even I could see that she didn't have a chance. You walk in, inject something into her vein, and in less than two hours she's well. It's eerie, it's spooky, it's frightening. It makes me doubt my sanity. You must have been tampering with things you never should have explored in the first place. You remind me of Faust after he signed the pact with the devil. He was a doctor, too, wasn't he? Marlowe called him Doctor Faustus."

"There's a difference between Doctor Faustus and me," said Keats. "He didn't have a license to practice medicine in the state of New York."

He watched her eyes carefully. Now he knew how the Salem housewives must have looked when they turned in their neighbors for witchcraft.

"My wife is just as grateful for all you have done as I am," said Mr. Rush. "She's just a little upset."

"But what was that medicine you injected into Nancy?" she asked.

"Something new," answered Keats.

"Doesn't it have a name?"

"No, just letters."

"Well, what are those letters? How do doctors refer to it when they are together?" Her voice had become shrill.

"They say F-U to each other."

"And what does 'eff you' mean?"

He laughed and shook his head. "Madam, I couldn't possibly tell you."

She colored and followed him to the front door.

"I agree that Nancy's recovery was miraculous," said Keats, turning to Mr. Rush. "But why give the devil the credit? If you tally up the number of miracles performed by the Lord compared to those performed by the devil, you'll find it's no contest. The Lord wins in straight sets." He turned to Mrs. Rush. "He shoots a sixty-four while Satan can't even make the cut."

"You certainly know the score, Doctor," said Rush. He added in an apologetic voice, "We're extremely appreciative, but we just can't figure out what hit us. It's like something out of science fiction."

"Not all the mysteries are in paperback," said Keats. "God saves a few for Himself."

A steady churchgoer, Rush boomed, "I'll buy that." He hesitated and then asked, "Do you think we'll be able to go to Easthampton next weekend?"

Keats laughed. "You'll go." He opened the door, enjoying the irony of the situation. He hadn't been to church in two years, but he had just helped God defeat the devil.

"One final question," said Mrs. Rush. "Is there anything we should be doing for Nancy?"

"Yes. Buy her a pair of pajamas with a neck opening three sizes too large."

He closed the door and rang the elevator bell.

5

WHEN KEATS came home a little after eight that evening, he found Annie Laurie in an unusually good humor. She had just received a substantial raise. Unlike most wives who become annoyed if their husbands are late for dinner, she never seemed to care what time he walked in. He got the impression that the longer he stayed away from her the happier she was. With the exception of his snoring, coughing, snuffling, and inability to earn much of a living, there was little about him that caught her attention. She had not even noticed that his cold and the warts on the back of his hand had simultaneously vanished. Since she felt that cooking a big meal that night would be too much for her after eight hard hours at the office, she served coffee and two sandwiches, which she had bought at the corner delicatessen. Afterward, they sat in the living room reading, he the *New York Times,* she the *Post.* When they were finished she tossed the *Post* to the couch on which he was sitting; he handed her the *Times.* Their marriage had been reduced to an exchange of newspapers.

Although he often had a desperate need to talk about his frustrations, he had learned not to tell her anything of his life, work, thoughts, or opinions. Quite early he had discovered that what she regarded as his long-winded speeches did not interest her. Later he could see that they irritated her. Nothing he said ever seemed to impress her. Tonight, he felt sure, he had news that would. He described in detail his experiences with the virus killer from the moment he opened Choate's door at the Medical Center a few days before until the moment he closed the Rushes' door tonight.

The first question she asked was, "How much do you have left?"

"Fourteen ml."

"And how many children would that cure?"

"Probably seven."

"By a stroke of luck you've got hold of one of the most valuable drugs ever invented. It's priceless. Where do you keep it?"

"In my little icebox in the lab."

"Is it labeled?"

"Yes, 'interferon.'"

She laughed. "That's smart. Nobody would ever catch on. You'll be rich in a year. The question is how much you should charge for a treatment. The city is filled with those noisy, little Mercedes 280s that sell for over ten thousand dollars each. In five years they're dented and dirty and look like hell. And they haven't made any money for the owner. A child, on the other hand, can work for forty years after he grows up. We've got the figures at the office. He can easily earn a million dollars during that time. Even a truck driver can earn half a million. A kid is worth a lot of money. And you can always count on the parents' love. There must be at least seven rich fathers in this country who would each give you thirty thousand dollars to save his child."

"Suppose a poor kid comes along?"

"See that he doesn't. If you gave your entire supply to ghetto children, how much more would you accomplish? You're concerned about depriving the poor. Don't the rich have feelings, too? Do you have the right to condemn seven children to death because their fathers earn money? Who do you think would get the drug in Russia, the porter's daughter or Brezhnev's grandson?"

"What do you want me to do? Auction it off as if I were a medical Parke Bernet?"

"That's just what I don't want you to do. I want you to look around and use some finesse. Tycoons' children are hit by viruses, too. If Wells had that drug, he'd make a fortune."

"He's a money machine."

"Is that so? He's thirty-eight, handsome, doesn't snore, has a flat belly, and runs the biggest pediatric practice in New York. So he's just a money machine. You, of course, are perfect, so perfect you can't make a living." Her voice softened. "If you would only wise up, I could give up my job. Then maybe things would be better between us."

"I'm going to inject the virus killer into any patient who needs it, first come, first served. I'm not going to deny it to the poor today so I can give it to the rich tomorrow. And I am not going to talk like a kidnaper. I'm not going to say to a parent, 'If you don't let me have thirty thousand dollars, you'll never see your child alive again.' "

She picked up her book. "No wonder you won't be the next director of Pediatrics. No brains and no guts." She stood up, walked to her room, and closed the door.

He should never have told her about the virus killer, he realized. He should have learned by now never to tell her anything. Maybe he was naive, but he expected a little praise and encouragement from his wife once in a while. Instead he always got a kick in the teeth. It took him two hours to go through a medical article that he would ordinarily have read in twenty minutes. Then he went to bed.

By a quarter to eight the next morning he had finished his examination of little Charlie Prince. The nurse reported that he had vomited three times during the night. Keats realized that he had forgotten an important piece of information, that he had missed a clue. Sins of omission were rarely forgiven in medicine. He remembered the nine-year-old girl from Queens whom the Princes had sent to him ten days before because the neighborhood doctor had been unable to make the diagnosis. She had a pink, pimply rash on her face, body, palms, and soles. Inside her mouth were many tiny erosions. He knew at once that he was dealing with a case of hand, foot and mouth disease, a condition caused by a Coxsackie virus. Although the little girl had made an uneventful recovery, others attacked by this agent were not so fortunate. It sometimes struck at the central nervous system. He recalled that she and Charlie had been inseparable companions. Now Charlie was vomiting, one of the early signs of meningitis, an inflammation of the coverings of the brain and spinal cord. Keats sighed and walked toward the elevator.

Coming toward him was Charlie's father, head of the fingerprint division of the New York City Police Department, who was everywhere known as "Finger" Prince, even though his first name was Michael.

"Have you been able to come up with anything yet, Doctor?"

"Charlie may have a Coxsackie virus infection. It's named after a town in the Catskills where it first appeared."

"Is it serious?"

"It is if it involves the central nervous system." Keats was careful not to use the words *brain* and *spinal cord*.

"He got it from his girl friend, didn't he?"

Keats, who hated to blame the other child, shrugged and said, "A lot of adults carry the virus."

After making two house calls he spent the rest of the day at his office. When he returned to Adams at four thirty he found that Charlie's condition had deteriorated. The boy had a stiff neck, a sign of irritation of the coverings of the brain and spinal cord. He had also lost the power of flexing his feet toward his shins. Captain and Mrs. Prince watched the examination with anxiety.

"I'm afraid there is involvement of the central nervous system," said Keats after he had herded them into the corridor. "I'm going to do a lumbar puncture to drain off a little spinal fluid for analysis."

"Is it painful, Doctor?" asked Mrs. Prince.

"I'll use a local anesthetic."

He went to the nurses' station, a fifteen-foot barricade behind which they answered the telephone, wrote reports, and had conferences. A dozen residents were arguing with and teaching each other. He walked up to the chief resident and said,

"Would you please do a spinal tap on a sick little boy of mine?"

The chief resident looked at his watch, shook his head regretfully, and said, "I'm sorry but I have to leave in a few minutes."

He was right. The great five-o'clock exodus would soon begin. Most of the residents were good family men. They had to go home to their wives and children. Those who were not were good family women. They had to go home to their husbands and children.

The chief resident beckoned to a first-year resident. "Do a spinal tap on the Prince kid." He turned to Keats and added, "He's on duty tonight."

The first-year resident who had graduated from medical school four months before and the fifty-four-year-old attending who had worked at Adams for thirty years walked along the corridor together.

"How many spinal taps have you done?" asked Keats.

"None," answered the resident, "but I've seen a lot."

"Do you think you can do this one? The boy is pretty sick."

"Of course I can. It's not open heart surgery, for chrissakes."

After they entered the treatment room Keats gave the resident a hard look. "I think I'll do this one myself. Watch me and I'll teach you some of the tricks."

In making this remark he knew that he was defying departmental policy. Lumbar punctures, chest taps, intravenous infusions, and blood transfusions were supposed to be performed by the house staff. For these procedures experienced attendings were expected to turn over their private patients to residents who often had had little experience. The senior men were told that the youngsters had come to Adams to do things themselves. If they were not permitted to, they would go to other hospitals. After all, they had to get something out of their residencies. The eighteen-thousand-dollar-a-year salary was never mentioned.

A nurse entered the treatment room with the lumbar-puncture set, which she unwrapped and placed on a small metal table. A moment later an older nurse wheeled Charlie in on a stretcher.

"You're going to stick a needle into my back, aren't you? Will it hurt?" asked the boy.

"I'll give you something so it won't," answered Keats. "There's just one thing. The nurse is going to bend your back. That may be uncomfortable."

"All right, but I can't move my feet anymore."

"I know."

While Keats scrubbed his hands and put on sterile rubber gloves the nurses carried Charlie from the stretcher to the long examining table. Then they took off his hospital gown and turned him on his side, with his back toward the pediatrician. Keats sat down on a stool just behind the boy and looked around.

"Where's the resident?"

"He said he had to make a telephone call," answered the older nurse.

Keats's jaw muscles tensed. He shook his head once. Then he used betadine solution to paint the lower half of Charlie's back, which he covered with a sterile lap sheet whose central, rectangular opening exposed the area on which he was about to work. As soon as he nodded to the nurse who faced him across the table she put one arm behind the patient's head, the other behind his knees, and bent them toward each other, thus separating the vertebrae so that the needle could slide in between them more easily.

"You'll feel a prick and then nothing," he said to Charlie.

With his left hand he palpated the projecting spinous processes which would act as his landmarks; with his right he injected procaine solution between the fourth and fifth lumbar vertebrae. After waiting several minutes to give the painkiller time to act, he pushed the four-inch needle with the sharp stylet inside through the hole the previous injection had made. When at last he felt some resistance, he pressed a little harder. There was a sudden give. He knew he was in the spinal canal. As soon as he pulled out the stylet, the other nurse held a test tube beneath the needle in Charlie's back to catch the crystal-clear fluid which was dripping from it. Keats almost wished the fluid had been cloudy. Turbidity would have been a sign of bacterial meningitis, a condition for which there were potent antibiotic remedies. He inserted the stylet, pulled out the needle with it, and applied a dressing.

"You were brave," he said as he shook Charlie's hand. "Now lie on your back."

The older nurse said, "I wish those boys would learn to do spinal taps like that."

When Keats returned at eight that night, the results of the spinal-fluid analysis were ready. The protein was markedly elevated but there were no cells. This combination, he knew, was characteristic of the dread Guillain Barré Syndrome, a rapidly ascending, symmetrical paralysis. Charlie had just fallen asleep. Captain and Mrs. Prince were standing in the corridor.

"The weakness in his feet is creeping up his legs," said Prince.

"I'm not surprised," said Keats. "He has an ascending paralysis, an uncommon condition which may be caused by toxins or viruses, including the Coxsackie virus."

"Can it hit all the muscles?" asked Prince.

"Yes, but let's hope it stops before it gets that far. Many children recover with complete return of muscle function."

"Is his life in danger?" asked Mrs. Prince.

Keats hesitated. "No, and it won't be unless the muscles of respiration become involved."

That night he slept very little. He kept returning to the thought that there were only seven doses of the virus killer left. He did not have the right to use it, he felt, unless a patient's life was threatened. The next morning he found that the paralysis had ascended to Charlie's waist. The lower extremities were limp, the reflexes had disappeared. But the boy was alert and cheerful. Case reports in the medical literature had indicated that children as badly involved as this had made excellent recoveries.

As Keats was leaving the floor, Dummer came up to him and said, "May I talk to you for a moment?"

They walked into the conference room and sat down. "I've just received a complaint about you," said the Director of Pediatrics. "I've been told that you took a lumbar tap away from a resident."

Keats gave a nasty laugh. "In the first place it was not a service case but a semiprivate patient of mine. Second, I asked the chief resident to do it, but he refused because it was too close to takeoff time. Third, the resident he assigned was a half-breed, a cross between a nitwit and a horse's ass. I didn't have a choice. I had to do the tap myself." He looked hard at his chief. "You know what goes on in this hospital as well as I do. The residents get a million and a half dollars a year. And who do you think pays it? The patients, of course. Much worse than that, there is often an unspoken agreement between the residents and the attendings to cheat the sick. A woman goes to a surgeon who agrees to take out her gall bladder for a thousand dollars. He sends her into Adams as his private or semiprivate patient. But he doesn't take out her gall bladder after she's put under anesthesia. Without her permission or her knowledge he lets the resident do the operation, which takes twice as long as it would have if he had done it himself. A couple of weeks later he sends a bill and pockets the check. The setup is a fraud. It's illegal."

"It's not illegal if the patient never finds out," said Dummer. "Besides, the surgeon is only an inch away from the resident."

"That's an inch too far."

Dummer went to the door, closed it, and came back to his seat. "I don't deny the truth of any of this," he said placatingly. "And I don't like it any more than you do. But you have to face the facts. In the hospitals today, the young people are leading the parade. Three years ago I decided to jump on their bandwagon. I've never regretted it. As a result, we have fourteen residents instead of two. And Bridge Wells, whose appointment was one of the greatest things that ever happened to the Department of Pediatrics."

"We would be better off with half as many residents."

"Not when it comes to prestige. A department is known by the number of residents it keeps. They're hard to get. And you can't get them if you don't understand them. They're in the driver's seat and they know it. They're demanding. They have no use for old men. They think we're responsible for Vietnam, corruption in government, pollution, crime, inflation, and everything else that's wrong with the world today."

"Maybe they're right. But the old men did some good things, too. We hit home runs with Babe Ruth and flicked the chalk lines with Big Bill Tilden. We abolished the sweat shops, pushed through the Wagner Act, and pulled the country out of its greatest depression. We started social security, welfare, and pensions for the old. We created the big unions and the big corporations. We were labor and management. We wiped out rickets and polio. We discovered penicillin and open heart surgery. We built boats to cross the Atlantic in five and a half days, and planes to do the job in five and a half hours. We jumped up and down on the moon and picked up a couple of rocks. But at least we got there. We voted for FDR and sent the boys to cross the Rhine—hell, we *were* the boys who crossed the Rhine. We raised the flag at Iwo Jima and cracked the Siegfried Line. We split the atom, and then wouldn't let the bastards blow up the world. They threw you in jail if you opened your mouth in Peking, Moscow, or Madrid. But nobody could take freedom of worship, freedom of the press, and freedom of speech from the people in this country while we were in our prime. And as long as we are alive, nobody ever will. We didn't bring on the Messiah, but at least we saw to it that most families—not all, unfortunately, but most—had three meals a day, a job, medical care, a car, a vacation, and braces on their children's teeth whether they needed them or not. We made some people happy, kicked a few asses, and didn't need to take drugs to screw a woman or go on living. I don't see the kids giving back any of the benefits we won for them. Let them ask themselves whether they can match our record."

Dummer rose and patted Keats on the shoulder. "Old-fashioned oratory is dead. Youth wants leaders who are cool. We have lots of residents now, thanks to Bridge Wells. I hope you won't do anything to antagonize them." He walked out, leaving the door open.

Keats waited a few moments before taking the elevator down to the main lobby. He was about to leave the building when Dr. Grant planted himself directly in his way. The sonofabitch was harder to run around than the Notre Dame line, said Keats to himself. He knew the Director of Laboratories as a fourth-rate scientist and a first-rate businessman. Some of the doctors did not agree with this assessment. They felt that Grant was a third-rate scientist. But everyone was of the opinion that he ran a good routine laboratory. Two years before, he had signed a five-year contract at a very low salary. In return for such apparent idealism he had asked the hospital to permit him to privately bill any patient an attending might send from his office to the Adams laboratory. The trustees and the administrator consented since they were not aware of the loyalty of the hospital doctors. Grant was. He knew that few of them ever used an outside laboratory. In 1972 his income was one hundred and four thousand dollars. The administrator tried to persuade him to negotiate a new contract. Grant said he would be delighted to in three years.

"May I speak to you for a moment?" he asked Keats. The question was rhetorical. "I understand you haven't been getting along too well with the house staff. You had a run-in with one of the new residents yesterday, didn't you?"

Keats wondered how he had found out so quickly. Then he remembered that if the wife of an Adams doctor missed a menstrual period, half the hospital knew about it the next day.

"It's a departmental matter," he said.

"It's a hospital matter," retorted Grant. "I'm chairman of both the committee on medical education and the residents' committee, and I can tell you that if word gets around that we don't treat our boys right, we won't have any new residents next year. Then all the departments will suffer, including mine."

Keats realized that Grant was creating this little scene so that he could discuss it with the members of the medical board when the applications for the position of director of Pediatrics were laid before them next month. He would undoubtedly contrast Wells's patron-saint relationship to the house staff with his own.

"Maybe you've got a point," said Keats diffidently. "I guess you must be an expert on medical education since you're being considered for the Le Bon Prize."

"I am? What is it?" asked Grant with considerable interest.

"Le Bon is Nobel spelled backwards. It's the Nobel Prize in reverse. It's given for the worst work in medicine instead of the best. Instead of your photograph, a negative appears in the newspapers, a costly process. Your biographical sketch is prepared not by a medical historian but by Cuddles Grosscunt, the madam of a famous whorehouse in Uppsala. Instead of inscribing your citation on ancient parchment, the authorities type it on toilet tissue. Instead of receiving seventy thousand dollars, you have to pay that sum to the Scandinavian committee. And you don't get to go to Sweden. They send two assassins over here who hang a fluorinated herring on your prick unless you write that check. 'Caries,' you're going to win the prize hands down."

This time he had no trouble getting past Grant.

He spent most of the day at his office seeing a few patients, answering the telephone, helping his secretary fill out school forms, and writing checks. Late that afternoon he returned to Adams. A careful neurological examination convinced him that Charlie's paralysis had not progressed. Maybe tomorrow it would begin to recede. Then he would not have to inject the boy with the virus killer. That would be better not only for the patient but for himself. Experimental drugs were not looked upon with favor at Adams. First the investigator had to obtain the approval of his chief. Keats smiled. Dummer, the cautious "Catabolic Kid," was a master of evasion, procrastination, and discouragement. He had destroyed more than one promising piece of research by his delaying tactics. He would be aghast at the tale of the virus killer. But even if he gave his consent to its use in an unbelievable burst of bold acumen, it could not be injected into a patient without the permission of the research committee, the pharmacy committee, and finally the seven-man medical board. For any medication to pass through this chain of command might take months, certainly weeks.

Keats too was interested in the safety of the virus killer. He realized that he had tried it on only two human beings and a dog. Chloramphenicol, a potent drug which had saved many lives, had been used on hundreds of thousands of people before the medical profession began to see that it was killing children by causing irreversible aplastic anemia. Suppose the virus killer proved lethal for the next patient? It was certainly not a substance to be used lightly.

If he ever decided that he was going to inject it into Charlie, he would certainly need the goodwill if not the active cooperation of Miss Starr, Supervisor of Nursing of the Department of Pediatrics. Nothing was ever done on the service without her approval. Dummer consulted her about everything. Wells was deferential, the nurses intimidated, and the members of the house staff actually respectful. Because of her regal stature and bearing they referred to her as the empress. Five foot eleven, one hundred and fifty-five pounds, with blonde hair, sky-blue eyes, and a beautifully proportioned, opulent figure, she was at fifty still a handsome woman. She touched up her few gray hairs not because she wished to appear young but because she felt that a mixture would have made her look unkempt. Once when Keats was walking along the corridor at a considerable distance behind her he passed a cluster of residents. One of them, fascinated by her hourglass figure, said,

"She must have been something in her day."

Keats stopped, hunched his shoulders the way he used to when the quarterback handed him the ball, and growled, "She's still something."

To his amazement she turned and gave him a dazzling smile.

This afternoon he decided that it would be wise for him to poke his head into her office and wave at her. Since Wells's schedules had banished the attendings from rounds, he had had little opportunity to talk to her. As he approached her office the floor nurses were standing at attention in front of her desk. She had just finished reprimanding them for their lackadaisical behavior.

"I did not ask you to sit down," she said, "because that is all you have been doing since I came in this morning. In the words of Noel Coward, your performance today can be described as a triumph of never-mind over it-doesn't-matter. You may leave."

He waited until the last nurse had left before entering her office.

"You must really want something," she said. "You haven't been here in three years."

"I haven't been to grand rounds in three years, either, not since the Wells-Dummer axis took over. I just wanted to find out if you still remembered me."

"You're so big you used to make me feel dainty when I stood next to you on grand rounds. A woman of my size doesn't forget a man like that so easily."

"You always make me feel the way I used to when I was carrying the ball for Columbia and the stands were roaring."

"Who was it who said that inside every thug there is a poet trying to get out?"

"You."

She laughed. "Are you still married?" Most people at Adams knew that he and his wife did not get along well.

He hesitated. "I guess you could say that." Then he waved at her, because that was why he had come, and walked away.

6

TRUDY STARR had entered the Adams Nurses' Training School directly from high school in 1940, when she was seventeen. In those days student nurses worked from seven A.M. to seven P.M. six days a week with three hours off every afternoon. In place of a salary they received free board, room, and education. Of the nine hours a day they spent on duty, three were devoted to lectures and six to assisting the graduate nurses and caring for the patients. In their third and final year, students were able to take over the functions of head nurses for brief periods, and often did. After graduation they rewarded Adams for feeding, sheltering, and educating them by working on the floors themselves for a modest salary. They rarely married before thirty. Their three-year training period had had only one purpose—to teach them how best to care for the sick. In 1962 the system was overthrown. The students disappeared from the floors. Their days were now taken up with lectures, seminars, discussions, demonstrations, and projects. Their education was no longer focused on the practical but on the academic. In 1971 the trustees abolished the nursing school, which was costing them almost two million dollars a year. They did so for two reasons. First, the students no longer took any part in the care of the patients. Second, soon after graduation most of them married, and, following their migrant husbands, settled down to work in local hospitals throughout the land. In other words, Adams was spending almost two million dollars a year to train nurses for every institution in the United States except itself.

The disappearance of the students was one of the main reasons why the nursing service, at least on the floors, so magnificent in the early forties, had become so miserable thirty years later. The hundreds of young girls who had once hurried along the corridors anxious to please, to serve, to make a good impression, had been replaced by a handful of graduates many of whom listened with one ear to the patients' buzzers and with the other to the sound of wedding bells. As soon as the latter became a reality, they rushed off to the hinterland on the arms of their husbands. There was a sense of impermanence about the staff. In 1973 the only way that a doctor could ensure adequate care for a sick adult was to persuade him to hire private nurses around the clock. To put him on floor care was to abandon him.

The deterioration in service was not caused by the young graduates themselves, most of whom were kind, hard-working, and intelligent, but by a new system created in the university centers by administrators. Formerly, a nurse had only one function—to take care of the sick. Now she had three: to write things down, to telephone, and to confer. Seated behind a fifteen-foot-long desk which served as a barricade, she spent one third of her time writing in charts, ledgers, and anything else that came to hand. One got the impression that the nursing office would not have objected if she had written on the floor or on the back of a coworker's white uniform. Unfortunately, she was like an unsuccessful author in that little of what she wrote was ever read. Another third of her time was spent telephoning, to whom or about what did not seem to matter. As long as she was seen talking into the mouthpiece, it was assumed that she was doing her duty. One embittered old surgeon said that the symbol of the nursing profession should be a woman in white looking a little like the Statue of Liberty but with a telephone receiver instead of a beacon in her raised hand. It was indeed hard to see how Florence Nightingale ever managed to survive without Alexander Graham Bell. The rest of a nurse's time was spent conferring with other nurses or with residents, probably deciding who would be on team A and who on team B that day. They rarely discussed a case with an attending. He was supposed to get his information from his patient's private-duty nurses. If the patient could not afford them, the attending learned little. Anyone on floor care who hoped to get a bedpan needed the cunning of a Ulysses, the power of a Stalin, and the appeal of a battered child. The demands of a full bowel or a distended bladder were considered secondary to those of an empty chart or an administrative conference. The seriously ill were sent to special intensive-care units.

Through the years Trudy Starr had watched her department abandon its original purpose, direct bedside nursing. When she graduated in 1943 at the age of twenty, the depersonalization process had not yet begun. She was one of the most brilliant students in her class; certainly the handsomest. The Directress of Nursing persuaded her not to join the Army Nursing Corps since Adams needed her at the moment, and would need her even more in the future. Two years later she was appointed head nurse in the infants' division; six years after that, Supervisor of Nursing of the entire Department of Pediatrics. No one so young had ever before held the position. The front office had confidence in her because she had shown herself to be a good administrator and something of a martinet. This confidence was not misplaced. She achieved a great success. After three years, however, she walked into the directress's office one morning and handed in her resignation, explaining that she was going to take a supervisory position in the prestigious Great Ormond Street Hospital for Children in London. Both her parents had died in 1945, she added. Adams was shocked and saddened. The Department of Nursing gave her a lovely tea.

For the next four years she wrote regularly to the directress. Every Christmas she sent cards to scores of people at the hospital. Then without warning she notified the nursing office at Adams that she had accepted a supervisory position at the *Kinderklinik* of the University of Heidelberg. She proved to be as diligent a correspondent from Germany as she had been from England. The hospital was to have another surprise, however. After having been at Heidelberg for three years, she appeared at eight one morning in the office of the Directress of Nursing and asked if she could have her old position back. The directress was delighted. The present supervisor was far from satisfactory. To a splendid record at Adams, Miss Starr had added seven years of service at two of the greatest hospitals in Europe. The American institution showed how far it had progressed during this time by giving her a cocktail party instead of a tea at the reception hall of the school of nursing. Most of the doctors and several of the trustees were there. In presenting her with a wristwatch on behalf of the hospital, Hexter, the administrator, unbent so far as to refer to her as the prodigal daughter.

In spite of the honors given her, she knew that there would be no place for her in the new world of nursing education. No one without a college degree would be allowed to hold an executive position. She enrolled at once in the School of General Studies of Columbia University. By attending night courses and summer sessions she obtained a B.S. in seven years. In 1973, when she was fifty, she already had twenty-one points toward her masters degree in nursing administration.

By this time she had become an Adams landmark, the bridge between the Gulbanian nursing school at the height of its glory and the ivory tower of the academicians at the height of theirs. She was the old and the new. Everyone agreed that pediatrics, intensive care, and the operating room gave the best nursing service in the hospital. She dressed with elegance, ran a small car, and lived in a lovely, rent-controlled three-room apartment in the East Seventies. A private income made little luxuries possible. When her father died in 1945, he left her forty thousand dollars' worth of gilt-edged securities. Twenty years later she sold them for one hundred and forty thousand dollars, half of which she put into tax-free municipal bonds, the rest into savings banks. To her prestige, efficiency, elegance, relative affluence and beauty was added an aura of mystery which made her even more attractive. No one at Adams had ever known anything about her private life. Then there were the pictures.

Guests who were invited to her home were stunned by the sight of the nineteen paintings which covered the walls. Many people regarded them as clever forgeries, having decided that the alternative was unthinkable. She cut short any questions about their provenance by changing the subject abruptly. But they were all originals. There were four Whistler's, three Sargent's, one Canoletto, three Monet's, two Pissaro's, three Turner's, and three Constable's. All depicted scenes of English life. She planned to leave them to the Tate in London provided they were kept together as the Trudy Starr collection. If this condition could not be met, then they would be given to some smaller British museum. They were not insured, first because she could not have afforded the premiums, and second because she was certain that no art thief would ever believe that an Adams nurse owned such a collection.

Although she had never married, nobody thought of her as a spinster, or a virgin either. Nevertheless, most of the people who worked at Adams would have been surprised, even shocked, to learn why she had so suddenly left the country in 1954. Two months before her departure, an Englishman walked into her office and asked if he might see a little girl who had just had her appendix removed. After giving her name, he explained that she was the daughter of an American friend. He reminded Miss Starr of a fencing foil, so slim and supple was he. He was sharp-featured, handsome, charming, and, as she later discovered, twenty years older than she. It was John Gloucester of the Foreign Service, one of the richest men in Great Britain. She took him to see the little patient, and then showed him the entire department, which he indicated was only of secondary interest to him. The following night he telephoned her. One week later they went to bed together at her apartment. Their seven-week affair proved even more delightful than they had anticipated. An expert in the arts of love to begin with, he gained strength from her youth and vitality. His wife in England was skinny, flat-chested, two years older than he, and rode to hounds. She was not, however, as sexually retarded as had been her grandmother, who like many another English bride had been told by her mother on her wedding day to grit her teeth and think of Queen Victoria whenever her husband made love to her. Mrs. Gloucester was much too modern to follow such advice. Whenever John had sexual intercourse with her she gritted her teeth and thought of King George the Sixth.

The week after Gloucester returned to England, he asked her over the telephone to come to London. With her background, he explained, she would have no trouble getting a supervisory position at the Great Ormond Street Hospital for Children. Her passport came with amazing speed. Two weeks after she had spoken to him she left the United

States. A supervisory position was indeed awaiting her at Great Ormond Street. The matron helped her find a little two-room flat in a quiet neighborhood. Miss Starr paid her own rent and all her other expenses. Every Wednesday evening at precisely seven thirty, Gloucester visited her. He left at precisely eleven thirty. He came even when she was menstruating. John Gloucester was a gentleman. She refused to accept anything from him except the single tickets to concerts, the opera, the ballet, and the theater he sent her so frequently. He insisted that she go everywhere unescorted. A chauffeured car that could not be traced to him took her to her destination, then called for her and took her home alone. He saw to it that she received regular dinner invitations to the homes of many of the most important people in Britain, leaders in the arts, the professions, industry, and finance. But he never took her anywhere himself. Too circumspect a man to risk a scandal, he preferred the secret and safe Wednesday-night assignations to a deeper relationship. If he made no mistakes, he might become Chancellor of the Exchequer some day. Miss Starr realized that hers was a Cupid and Psyche affair. The god crept into her bed protected by the darkness of the night and left before the sun could identify him. But her work at the hospital was fascinating, her social life dazzling, and her sexual needs fulfilled. She was content. Every year on her birthday he sent her an oil painting. At first she did not know how much they were worth. When she did, it was too late for her to refuse them. Besides, since she had no intention of ever selling them, they had no monetary value for her.

After she had enjoyed London for four years, Gloucester informed her one Wednesday night that the Foreign Service was transferring him to Bonn. He suggested that she move to nearby Heidelberg. A supervisory position would await her at the *Kinderklinik* of the University, he was sure. She moved at once. She liked her new position as much as the old. Language was no barrier since her maternal grandmother had taught her German as a child. Occasionally she would fly to London for a weekend party. The chauffeured limousine always called for her at the hotel and took her back alone. The seven-thirty Wednesday-evening secret meetings at her apartment were meticulously continued. But since he had to drive back to Bonn, they were terminated at precisely ten thirty.

Only once in the seven years she spent in Europe did he take her out. One Saturday in the spring, he telephoned her from Bonn to ask her to go with him to Schwetzingen the following morning. His wife was spending a week in London. He could not call for Trudy at her apartment, of course. In broad daylight? Unthinkable. Nor at the Europaischer Hof, Heidelberg's finest hotel. That would be political suicide. He preferred an obscure trolley stop at the outskirts of town.

He had dressed inconspicuously in an effort to mask his eye-catching elegance. During the ride they did not speak to each other. Should anyone recognize him, he could make believe that he did not know her. Miss Starr had ridden in trolleys as a little girl. She had always felt they were as peculiar to the city as skyscrapers. This one was different. For half an hour it traveled at break-neck speed over farm land, fields, and meadows. When it reached the vast ducal estates, she could see clouds of white lilacs towering over the gates inside. On boards set up on trestles outside, crowds of Germans were eating the white asparagus for which Schwetzingen was equally famous. As the English aristocrat and the American nurse walked along the perfect lawns of the estate, he kept ten feet away from her so that if an acquaintance should greet him he could turn his back to her as if they had not come together. She realized that this outing represented a sacrifice for so cautious a man. After a few minutes, when he became convinced that no disgrace awaited him, he walked by her side. They looked at the great fountains and the little ones, the gleaming white stone statues of stags and stallions, the palaces and the summer houses. They walked over the narrow, arched bridges and through the tiny man-made forests. They had white asparagus for lunch in a dim corner of a restaurant on the grounds where no one was likely to see them. In the afternoon he took her to a spacious house next to a mosque. It was here, he explained, that the duke kept his beloved mistress. She was Turkish, and, being a woman of exquisite morality, wept because she had no place in which to pray. He had built her the mosque, which was still the only one in Germany. The duchess, a good Lutheran, was enraged at the double humiliation of having a mistress and a Muhammadan place of worship on her estate. In the eighteenth century, however, there was little a wife could do. She did persuade the head gardener to sow the grounds around the mistress's house with onions, and to use a heavy hand. In the summer the stench was overpowering. Even two hundred years later, Miss Starr could smell a faint odor. To her amazement, Gloucester motioned her to conceal herself behind a dazzlingly white stone stallion while he looked around to be sure no one was watching them. Then, popping a mint into his mouth so that she would never associate his kiss with the smell of onions, he touched her lips gently with his. On the way home, he told her that this little spree would have to last them a lifetime. He kept his word. He never took her out again.

At the end of her third year at Heidelberg, she remembered her grandmother's favorite proverb, which was *zu viel ist ungesund,* "too much is unhealthy." She handed her resignation to the *Oberschwester* at the *Kinderklinik,* who shook her head in disbelief and wiped her eyes. Two weeks later, on a Wednesday evening in the spring, she led Gloucester into her little dining alcove where the table was covered with white asparagus and white lilacs. They had such a good time in bed that night that he did not leave until five minutes after eleven. He did not know it at the time but he was never to see her again. The following afternoon she took the plane from Frankfurt to New York. The next morning she telephoned to thank him for the part he had played in making her stay in England and Germany so enjoyable. She asked him not to write or telephone her. He never did. John Gloucester was a gentleman.

He did, however, send her an oil painting on every one of her birthdays. She knew he missed her because the masterpieces kept getting more costly and more magnificent. Each year she sent him a letter telling him everything about her reactions to the pictures and nothing about herself. He never answered her. At seven o'clock one morning in 1973, twelve years after she had left Heidelberg, his confidential secretary telephoned her. He was seventy-three with moderate nerve deafness, early cataracts, and a paralysis of one vocal cord. He heard no evil, saw no evil, and spoke no evil; and very little that was good, either. In his hoarse voice he informed her that Gloucester had died an hour before. She flew to London for the funeral. No one knew who she was. She returned that night. Even in death John Gloucester was a discreet man. He left her nothing.

In 1967 she had had another affair, this time with a much finer man. He was her own age, and neither married nor betrothed, except perhaps to death. At their first meeting he told her that he had Hodgkins disease, but that the doctors had said that X-ray treatments and chemotherapy could preserve his life indefinitely. They were wrong. He did well for two years. Then his condition began to deteriorate. Formerly a busy architect, he could no longer keep up with his assignments. His savings dwindled. One day he confessed to her that he could no longer afford to stay in his apartment. He would have to move, he knew not where. She went to the office of a prominent real estate operator whose little daughter's life had been saved at Adams by expert surgery and good nursing care. More than once he had assured her that whenever any of his apartments became vacant, he would be glad to rent them to Adams's nurses. This was something different, she explained to him. She wanted him to draw up a one-year lease at an absurdly small sum for an architect who was dying of Hodgkins disease. She would write a check for the difference at once. When she handed her lover the lease, she informed him that it was for a rent-controlled apartment and was the bargain of the century. It was fortunate that he was fond of his new home because he became bedridden in six months. She hired an elderly woman to cook for and take care of him, explaining to him that she was working for room and board. She herself nursed him whenever she was not on duty at the hospital. Just before he died, he wrote out the monthly check for the landlord in a surprisingly firm hand. Then he smiled at her and said,

"See, I'm not a pauper. The rent is paid."

She had not slept with a man since.

When Keats waved to her as he left her office later in the afternoon, she knew he had not told her the real reason for his visit. The charm under those old football bones was concealing something deeper, something, she felt, that concerned his patient with the Guillain Barré Syndrome. She walked into Charlie's room. He seemed alert and cheerful. He could move his arms easily. He had no trouble breathing. In hospital jargon his condition was stable. But she slept fitfully that night. The first thing she did when she arrived at Adams at seven thirty the next morning was to hurry to his room. She was appalled. He was lying on his back gasping with mucus dripping from his mouth.

She patted him on the shoulder. "You don't have to be frightened anymore. We'll all take care of you now."

She rushed to the barricade. Behind it there were three nurses. Two were telephoning and one was writing in a chart.

80

"Why aren't you with the Prince boy?" Miss Starr asked, trying to control her anger. "Have you notified Dr. Keats or a resident?"

The chart writer stood up. "Why? Is anything wrong with Charlie? We had four admissions last night, and we have to get the reports ready for the day shift."

"Four admissions!" exclaimed Miss Starr. "In World War II a troop train would unload two hundred and sixty patients at a time on a general hospital. What would you have done? Given up?" She looked hard at the two who were on the telephone. "I want you to put Charlie in an oxygen tent this minute."

"Without a doctor's order?" asked one in amazement.

"Without a doctor's order," replied the supervisor. "And stay with the patient. Then, if you can't think of anything to do, pray. But don't use the phone. God won't be on the other end of the line."

She went to her office and called Keats at his home. "Charlie Prince is terribly sick. He's in respiratory failure. I took the liberty of putting him in an oxygen tent without first asking for your permission. I hope you're not angry."

"I'm grateful," said Keats. "I'll be over as soon as I can throw on some clothes."

He had just finished taking a shower. He did not wait to shave or have breakfast. On the way down in the elevator he glanced at himself in the mirror. He certainly did not look like New York's best-groomed man. The sight of Charlie lying in the tent shocked him. The examination was brief. The boy's lips were blue even in fifty-percent oxygen. His upper extremities were now paralyzed, and the muscles of respiration so weakened that he had to struggle to breathe. An appealing look in his eyes made Keats bend down and put his ear close to the patient's lips.

"I can't swallow," said Charlie in a horrible, gurgling voice. "I can't move anything. And I can't breathe very well. Is that the way you feel just before you die?"

Keats straightened up. "You're not going to die," he said gruffly. But he was far from sure.

He walked rapidly to Miss Starr's office, driven by a sense of guilt. He should have given Charlie the virus killer yesterday, he now realized. If he gave it to him now, it would take at least an hour for it to act. The boy would be dead by then unless he could keep him breathing. And the drug, whatever it was, couldn't revive the dead.

As he entered Miss Starr's office she handed him the telephone like a good operating-room nurse anticipating a surgeon's demand for an instrument.

"Will you get a respirator here at once, please," he said to her.

She walked to the barricade. The day shift had just arrived. A pretty nurse, a telephone receiver pressed to her ear, was smiling broadly.

"Hang up at once, please," said Miss Starr sharply. The girl hung up.

In the office, Keats was dialing the operating room. Luckily Airov, the Director of Anesthesiology, answered the telephone.

"I have an eleven-year-old boy with the Guillain Barré Syndrome on the seventh floor," said the pediatrician. "He not only has a paralysis of all four extremities, but of his diaphragm and abdominal muscles as well. He's in acute respiratory failure. Unless I can get him hitched to a respirator, he's going to die in the next few minutes. Could you send someone down to put in an endotracheal tube?"

"I'll come down myself," said Airov in what his wife called his beautiful brogue. Although he had come to the United States forty years before, he had never lost his virile Russian accent. His enemies claimed that he practiced ten minutes in front of a mirror every morning to preserve it.

When Keats returned to Charlie's room two technicians from the inhalation-therapy service were wheeling in the Bennett MA 1, a third-generation volume respirator which they immediately connected to an oxygen line in the wall. This sophisticated machine pushed into the lungs a prearranged, unchanging volume of an air-oxygen mixture with each inspiration whether the resistance in the bronchial tubes was great or small. Since the average person sighs five times an hour, the machine sighed five times an hour, too, in order to prevent any tiny areas in the outlying portions of the lungs from collapsing. The head technician set the volume at four hundred ml. for each inspiration; the respiratory rate at eighteen per minute. Airov strode into the room with a laryngoscope wrapped in a sterile towel in his hand. He was a massive, handsome man with gray hair and gentle hands. Without a word from him the nurses wheeled the oxygen tent away. After stroking Charlie's cheeks and quickly explaining what he was about to do, the anesthetist depressed the patient's tongue with the laryngoscope and slipped the endotracheal tube into his windpipe. It took him but a moment to pick up a syringe and inject some air into the little balloonlike collar around the tube. This maneuver was designed to prevent any leakage of oxygen later on. The final step was to connect the endotracheal tube to the respirator. Immediately the machine began to breathe for a boy who soon would not be able to breathe for himself. Airov and Keats watched Charlie's lips. When they turned pink, the two men walked to the door.

"Bad, huh?" said the anesthetist.

Keats nodded.

Captain and Mrs. Prince had just arrived. The pediatrician took them aside, explained exactly what had happened to their son and what was now being done for him. Following this, he guided them to a corner of the corridor where he would not be overheard.

"I've recently injected a new medication into three patients with remarkable results." He did not tell them that one of the patients was a dog. "It's experimental, though, so I have to get your permission to use it on your son."

"You have it, you have it!" cried Captain Prince.

Keats crossed the bridge to the research building. Tugend was hovering in the hall. After giving the spy a nasty look, he walked into his laboratory. The dog jumped up and began to lick his hand. He should have taught it to bite Tugend on command, he decided. After hesitating for a moment while he thought over the dosage, he transferred two ml. from the bottle in the refrigerator to a sterile tube.

He walked into Miss Starr's office and closed the door.

"I'm going to ask a favor of you. Would you help me give an intravenous injection to the Prince boy? I should have given it to him yesterday."

"I don't do bedside nursing anymore. I have younger and prettier girls for that."

"Younger, yes. Prettier, no."

She smiled and stood up. They walked rapidly to the patient's room. To her surprise, Keats asked the Princes and the three nurses to leave. While he drew the virus killer into a syringe, she removed the boy's hospital gown, rubbed alcohol on the bend of his left elbow, applied a tourniquet to his arm, and steadied his forearm. As soon as the pediatrician slid the needle into the vein, she released the tourniquet. A second later he emptied the virus killer into the bloodstream. He pulled out the needle at once. After making sure that there would be no bleeding from the puncture site, he guided her to the other end of the room.

"I'd be grateful if you didn't mention what I've just done," he said softly. "Forget it, put it from your mind, make believe it never happened."

"How can I do that? It would not only be against the rules, but sloppy nursing, which is even worse. I simply have to record this injection."

He put his hands in the side pockets of his white coat. "I guess you do. The trouble is that I've injected an experimental drug, and I'm not supposed to do that without getting the permission of Dr. Dummer, two committees, and the medical board. There just wouldn't have been enough time. Besides, the big brass would never have allowed me to go ahead."

"What did you inject?"

"You won't believe me, but I don't know."

"What is it supposed to be?"

"Interferon."

"All right, how about this? I'll write in the nurses' notes that you injected two ml. of an interferon solution. The nurses' notes are so filled with stereotyped phrases, clichés, and unimportant information that nobody ever bothers to read them. You can write on the doctors' progress sheet whatever you want. I'm familiar with your handwriting. The only man in the country who would be able to read your note would be the cryptographer who cracked the Japanese naval code in World War II. Your secret will be safe."

He smiled. "It's a deal."

"Do you expect Charlie to react badly to the drug?"

"On the contrary, I expect him to be well in three hours."

"Doctor, Doctor!" She smiled. "But it's a lovely, sentimental idea anyway."

They walked along the corridor to the spot where the Princes were standing. The nurses streamed back into the room.

"If this drug works the way I hope it will," said Keats, "you may see an unbelievable improvement in a very short time. Should that happen, I don't want you to think that I've been dabbling in black magic or that I'm in league with the devil."

"It should only happen," said Mrs. Prince.

"Doctor," said the captain, putting his arm around his wife, "we're Catholics. We believe that no miracle is too great for the Lord."

Keats returned to the room with the Princes and sat by Charlie's bed. From time to time Miss Starr came in to check the respirator. It was working perfectly. The boy's lips remained pink. In half an hour the mucus stopped dripping from his mouth. He could now swallow. In an hour he began to move his arms, in an hour and a half his lower extremities. In two hours Keats noticed that he was breathing on his own and not in synchronization with the respirator. He was overriding the machine. The pediatrician went to Miss Starr's office and telephoned the operating room. Airov had just finished giving the anesthesia for a tonsillectomy.

"You can come down now and remove the endotracheal tube," said Keats.

"You must be out of your mind," retorted the anesthetist.

"Come down and see."

Airov was in the room in five minutes. He observed Charlie carefully for a moment and then disconnected the tube from the respirator. Charlie's breathing was normal. After watching him for a quarter of an hour, Airov deflated the balloonlike cuff and quickly removed the endotracheal tube from his windpipe. There were no respiratory difficulties. The patient, though slightly hoarse from the irritation of the tube, breathed as well as he ever had. Airov watched him for a few more minutes and then walked to the door. Captain and Mrs. Prince stood dumbfounded at the other end of the room.

The anesthetist turned to Keats and said, "We both must be out of our minds." Then he walked to the elevator, shaking his head from time to time.

Keats went to the cafeteria on the third floor and had a big breakfast. On his way back to see Charlie he stopped at Miss Starr's office.

"How about admiring my lovely, sentimental idea?"

They walked to the patient's room side by side. Once their arms touched. Miss Starr thought back to the day she had strolled along the lawns of Schwetzingen with John Gloucester ten feet away. Charlie was sitting up in bed.

"How do you feel?" asked Keats.

"I haven't felt this well since I was a kid," said the patient.

His parents and the nurses laughed. They would have laughed at anything he said.

"I want you to walk around the room with your hands raised," said Keats.

The boy obeyed.

"Now lower your arms and hop on your right foot. Now on your left," said his doctor.

The boy performed the tasks perfectly.

"You've been a wonderful patient," said Keats. "Your name should be reversed. Instead of Charlie Prince, it should be Prince Charlie, Bonnie Prince Charlie after another brave young man who almost became King of England. You can't become King of England because you're an American Catholic. But you could become a king in some other field, like medicine."

Charlie, who was wise in the ways of the police department, said, "When the time comes, will you write me a letter to that effect?"

"If I'm alive, I'll write you the letter," said Keats. "If I'm dead, I'll smile up at you from hell."

Charlie was shocked. "Hell!" he shrieked. "If they make a mistake like that, my father will go to the Cardinal."

"Don't you worry," said Mrs. Prince. "There's a seat in heaven reserved for the doctor next to St. Luke, the Beloved Physician."

Keats bowed and guided Miss Starr through the door. As they walked along the corridor, he said,

"Well, that's the end of my sentimental journey."

She smiled and put her hand on his arm. "Maybe it's just the beginning."

That afternoon Dummer visited her. "What's this I hear about a miracle worker on my service?" he said with considerable irritation. "A boy on the respirator with paralysis of all four extremities was reported to have been cured in a couple of hours. What did Keats inject into him? Something from outer space? Or is the whole thing just a lot of talk?"

Seated behind her desk, Miss Starr stifled a feigned yawn. "Excuse me. I didn't sleep very well last night."

Dummer eyed her beautiful torso. I'll bet you didn't, he said to himself. Or at least very much.

"Dr. Keats gave two ml. of an interferon solution," she said in a matter-of-fact voice.

Dummer, who did not know what interferon was, looked knowledgeable and said, "I see. That explains a lot."

As she was leaving the building at five thirty that afternoon, she felt a tap on her shoulder.

"May I drive you home?" asked Keats. "Or would you prefer not to be seen with an unshaved roughneck?"

She hesitated. Her car was on the other side of the street. "I'd love to sit next to a rough and healthy man for a change," she said at last.

He realized that she had been thinking out loud so he remained silent as they walked to his car. Opposite her apartment house was a parking space which he slid into automatically with a grim smile. He would have taken a legal parking place anywhere, even if it were in front of the gates of hell.

"Won't you come up for a drink?" she asked. "You've had a nerve-wracking day."

"I'd come up even if I hadn't."

The quiet elegance of her apartment relaxed him at once.

"What will you have to drink?" she asked.

"A screwdriver."

She walked into the kitchen. In a moment he heard the whir of a machine. She was evidently making his drink with fresh orange juice. He began to examine the pictures, methodically attempting to read the signatures. When she entered with the drinks, he turned and said,

"They're real, aren't they?"

She nodded.

"How did you ever acquire such a collection?" he asked.

"I never talk about my pictures."

"I didn't mean to pry. It's simply that you've got an unbelievable exhibition here."

"No more unbelievable than the exhibition you put on this morning with your interferon solution."

They sat down. She sipped her Canadian Club and ginger ale. He gulped his screwdriver noisily.

"I'll tell you how I acquired the pictures," she said, "if you tell me the story of your magic interferon solution. Is it a deal?"

He shook his head. "No. It wouldn't be fair. You don't want to tell me about your pictures. But I want to tell you about the virus killer. In fact, if I don't, I think I'll blow a gasket."

He told her everything. How he had picked up the solution at the Medical Center from an old classmate, the illustrious Professor Choate, who had assured him that it was pure interferon. How he had cured a dying dog. How he had injected the material into his own vein. How the virus killer had saved the lives of Nancy Rush and Charlie Prince. And finally how his wife had branded him as brainless and gutless because he would not capitalize on its profit-making possibilities.

"One thing is certain," he concluded. "Whatever the drug is, it's not interferon."

"You're a wonderful man, whatever the drug is. You've saved two lives that no one else in the world could have saved. You've cured the poor dog. And you didn't do so badly for yourself. You got rid of your nasty cold."

He smiled. "And my warts."

"Oh, I never minded them."

"That's because I never touched you."

"I wouldn't have minded that either." She sipped her drink. "It must have taken a lot of courage to inject yourself and those two children with an unknown drug. It's you who are the virus killer. You must be a happy man."

He finished his drink. She saw that he wanted to talk so she did not offer to get him another.

"I'm not happy," he said.

Her eyes widened. "Why do you say that?"

He seemed embarrassed. "It's an unpleasant topic." He shook the ice in his glass. "My wife hasn't gone to bed with me in three years. When that happens to a man of fifty-four, he loses the knack. His reflexes go."

She couldn't help smiling. What a lover, the poor man! she said to herself. But out loud she said, "The Sioux Indians have a legend about Hooaptee, god of the sunshine and of the thunder clouds, who was so disconsolate at the death of his beloved wife that for ten years he wandered over the earth without looking at a woman. On his return, he saw a goddess from the land of the sky-blue water and lusted after her. For one hundred days and one hundred nights they lay on the ground and made love to each other. They thrashed and they pounded, they squirmed and they shook, and their powerful up-and-down movements drove them deeper and deeper into the earth. On the hundredth night they fell asleep exhausted in each other's arms. When they awoke the next morning they were lying in sun-spangled, sky-blue water. Soft-mouthed little fish were nibbling at their toes.

They sat up and looked around them to see what their lovemaking had accomplished. They were impressed. They had created the Grand Canyon." She finished her drink. "Hooaptee was a thousand years old and had gone without a woman for ten years. You're only fifty-four and haven't made love in three. For a virile man like you, three years' abstinence is just a comma in the punctuation of sex. Someday you'll be young again. You may not dig yourself a second Grand Canyon, but you'll end up with a creditable furrow."

He smiled. "Only with the girl from the land of the sky-blue water. The land may not exist, but the girl certainly does. May I come here again?"

"I'll be disappointed if you don't."

He stood up. When they reached the door he took her hand and kissed it. Then he walked down five flights of stairs because he did not want anyone in the elevator to see the expression on his face.

She stood facing the door. Another walk down a dead-end street, she said to herself. I'm fifty and I've never had a marriage to my name, not even a bad one. I've always had to share a man with a wife or a disease. I've held thousands of children in my arms, but never my son or daughter. I specialize in inaccessible men, men preempted by marriage or hopeless illness. In the end all I have is a museum in my home. Oh, but that isn't fair. It hasn't been all emptiness. There have been some good things, too. I've had my work, seven exciting years in England and Germany, and one nice afternoon in Schwetzingen. And I helped a good man die with his chin up.

She walked to the couch and sat down. If Jim Keats gets that thirty-five-thousand-dollar-a-year job, she continued to herself, maybe I can make him take me to Schwetzingen. I know just how it will be. We'll have breakfast together at the Europaischer Hof. He'll growl at a waiter because he thinks he's a Nazi. Later he'll offer to punch some German in the mouth because he looked at me twice, but the man will walk away. In the trolley car he'll sit with his arm around me, perspiring and talking in a loud voice. The passengers will all stare at him, fascinated by his size, his tough face, and his bent football nose. When we reach the ducal estate we'll walk close to each other along the beautiful lawns. He'll hold my hand as much for his protection as for my own. As soon as we reach the mistress's mosque, I'll tell him the story about the onion fields. He'll smile. And he won't pop a mint into his mouth. He'll just take me in his arms and kiss me in front of a hundred astounded Germans. Then he'll sweat a little and worry about his reflexes.

She cooked herself a minute steak, which she ate with a simple salad. Afterward, she read the *American Journal of Nursing*. When she walked into the bedroom at ten o'clock, she was smiling. For the first time in nineteen years she had not looked at her pictures.

7

THE REMARKABLE cure that Keats had just accomplished did not bring him the satisfaction he had anticipated. Twelve ml. of the virus killer remained, enough to save the lives of six children who without it would die. But what of the other sixty million in the country all of whom were susceptible to viral infections? Since the medication would soon be exhausted, it would never have existed as far as they were concerned. Like man himself, it would come up in a day and vanish in a day. Keats felt like the pediatrician who was supposed to have been offered three wishes by a genie. Being something of a saint, the doctor had replied, "I would like to use each wish to save the life of a child." After his request had been granted and he had received the written thanks of the parents together with six insurance forms which he was asked to fill out in duplicate within seven days, the genie, according to the story, appeared before him again, this time reportedly swirling out of a vial of penicillin.

"Well, schmuck," said the supernatural being, "what are you going to do now? You're back where you started from."

"I guess I'll have to put an ad in the *New York Times* for another genie."

"Not a bad idea. But remember, if you're lucky enough to get a second chance, choose a wish with a future."

That was the trouble with the virus killer, Keats mused. It had no future. It certainly was not pure interferon. In fact its formula was unknown. Until it was determined, the medication could not be duplicated. His duty was clear. He would have to return the entire batch to Choate at the Medical Center for analysis.

The morning that Charlie Prince was discharged from the hospital Keats arrived at his office fifteen minutes late.

"Professor Choate's secretary has telephoned three times so far," his receptionist informed him. "She is frantic. I thought that scientists were supposed to be cool, calm, and collected, and that their attitudes rubbed off on the help."

"Choate is about as cool, calm, and collected as a one-armed paperhanger with the itch trying to wind a Waterbury watch. He's got a lot on his mind. What did he want?"

"His secretary wouldn't tell me. I promised that you would be at the Medical Center at two this afternoon."

When Keats entered Professor Choate's office at precisely two o'clock the virologist rose, inclined his head toward an old man seated next to his desk, and said, "Dr. Keats, Mr. Wright, the trustee."

The old man rose, too. "*A* trustee, Dr. Keats. There are thirty-four others. The reason why your friend calls me *the* trustee is that I contribute more than any of the rest, especially to his department. If I should become remiss in my donations next year, he would substitute the indefinite for the definite article."

As soon as the three were seated, Choate turned to Keats. "Did you squirt my so-called interferon up the noses of your little patients?"

"No."

Choate slumped in the chair behind his untidy desk. "True scientists are supposed to be unbelievers, but I am going to say thank God just the same. What did you do with it?"

"I injected it intravenously."

Choate straightened up at once. "You're driving me back to atheism. I specifically told you not to give it intravenously. Don't you realize that we are all responsible for whatever happened, not only you and I but my department and the Medical Center as well? Did any of the children die?"

"Nobody died. Now tell me why you are so disturbed."

"All right. The material I gave you under the impression that it was pure interferon was nothing of the sort. The technician who prepared it is a hopeless schizophrenic. I have just come from visiting him at the psychiatric hospital. He is hallucinating, incoherent most of the time, and suffering from bizarre delusions. He will never recover. From a few remarks he has made in less confused moments and from the accounts of eyewitnesses, I think I can reconstruct what he did during the two hours before he brought the solution into this office. He must have poured most of the interferon down the sink. Then he evidently removed small amounts of viruses, liquids, enzymes, chemicals, and a variety of other substances, thirty-six in all, from every laboratory in the building, and added them to your interferon bottle. I say thirty-six because thirty-six pairs of once-sterile gloves were found in the trash basket outside the positive-pressure room. We will never know what these substances were because he replaced the original containers in the exact positions in which he found them. Finally he took the brew, which even if he should recover he could never duplicate, and had it irradiated by the linear accelerator. Now do you understand why I am disturbed?"

Mr. Wright crossed his legs. "The Medical Center assumes no responsibility for untoward reactions caused by the unauthorized use of medications prepared in its laboratories. However, if children have been hurt, I will pay for a reasonable out-of-court settlement."

Keats smiled. "Dr. Choate has no reason to be disturbed and every reason to be gratified. Without realizing it, he has not only saved the lives of two children and a dog, but rid me of a persistent cold and a cluster of unsightly warts."

In the greatest detail he told them the story of the virus killer, omitting only those portions which had to do with his wife's reactions.

Choate seemed stunned.

Wright uncrossed his legs. "I am sure every word is true. I am not skeptical. But I am surprised to hear a fairy tale in a scientist's office."

"Where else would you hear one today?" asked Keats. "When I was in medical school, Rh disease, which had just been recognized as a clinical entity, killed sixty percent of the newborns it attacked. Many of the survivors were brain damaged. Ten years later exchange transfusions reduced the mortality to two percent and none of the survivors were brain damaged. Today, the Rh negative mother who receives a small injection of RhoGam within seventy-two hours after each delivery will give birth to a normal baby every time. Within my medical lifetime Rh disease has been discovered, cured, and finally abolished. That's a fairy tale. Scientists are beating Hans Christian Andersen at his own game."

"They are doing it every day with open heart surgery, antibiotics, and scores of other discoveries," added Choate. "And may I remind you that this laboratory has a few accomplishments to its credit—thanks to your generosity, Mr. Wright."

"By George," said the old trustee, "I believe you have written your fairy tales on the backs of my checks." He smiled. "I am delighted to have been your publisher."

Keats reached down into his little black bag, brought out the bottle containing the virus killer, and placed it on the desk in front of Choate.

"Bill, I'm returning what's left of the magic brew so that you can analyze it, reproduce, and, I hope, soon turn it over for manufacture."

Choate gave a bitter laugh. "When it comes to pure science you are a babe in the woods. There isn't one chance in ten thousand that I could make your fantasy come true."

"What's the matter, don't you have the equipment?"

"You know we do. We have everything from abacuses to computers. Maybe even brains. If we run short of those, I can go to my friends at Rockefeller University, where they have wall-to-wall Nobel Prize winners. But, unfortunately, we have something else. We have our limitations. Sure, I can analyze the stuff and tell you how much carbon, nitrogen, oxygen, hydrogen, and sulfur it contains. But what good would that do? Have you any idea how much time and effort it took to discover the formulae of insulin, thyroxin, and pituitary-growth hormone? Battalions of eminent scientists worked on them for years. And most important of all, the raw material could be constantly replenished—from the pancreas, the thyroid, and the pituitary of pigs and cattle." He looked at the bottle in front of him. "Those biochemists didn't have to work with a lousy twelve ml. that can never be replaced. When we've run through this where can we get more? This solution probably consists of hundreds of organic compounds, many as yet unknown and all of unbelievable complexity. Which one is the virus killer? Or is it the result of the constant interaction of dozens of substances each of which must be added in a certain sequence and be present in a fixed amount? How stable is this solution? How soon will it disintegrate and lose its potency?"

He pushed the bottle gently across the desk. "Shoemaker stick to your last. Take it back to Adams and save six more lives."

Keats laid the bottle in front of Choate again. "What are six lives compared to the hundreds of thousands you could save if you hit the jackpot? Who knows better than you that cancer may be caused by viruses?"

"Gentlemen," interrupted the old trustee, "in this debate you seem to have switched roles. Dr. Keats, the clinician, the bedside doctor, the man with the little black bag, is prepared to sacrifice six children on the altar of science. Dr. Choate, the pure scientist, is prepared to give up the chance of making the discovery of the century in order to save them. I find this very strange."

"It's not so strange," said Choate. "I know a famous and tremendously successful psychoanalyst who envies lowly general practitioners because they visit patients in their homes and in hospitals while he himself is chained to his seat nine hours a day. I feel much the same way. Many is the time I have threatened to steal a stethoscope, storm out of my laboratory, and treat the sick. People, when you get to know them, are more interesting than viruses, although in some cases, I'm forced to admit, the comparison turns out to be pretty close. On the other hand, Dr. Keats, who has devoted his life to treating children, spends most of his free time in his little laboratory at Adams. He is a scientist manqué."

Mr. Wright nodded. "Excellent. Both of you are striving to become the complete physician, or, to paraphrase Izaak Walton, the 'Compleat Angler.' Both of you are fishing, not for souls like St. Peter, but for lives."

There was a long silence.

"What would you do with the contents of the bottle?" Keats asked the trustee at last.

"I propose the Solomon solution," answered the old man. "Cut the baby in half."

The two doctors looked at each other. Then they both nodded. Choate rose. "This time I'm going to handle things myself." He took the bottle and left the room. Fifteen minutes later he returned with a smaller bottle, which he handed to Keats. "Here are six ml. of you know what. I certainly don't."

"Dr. Choate," said the old trustee, "if you need financial support to get this project started, call on me. It is as good a cause as any that is available to me. At seventy-five I can't spend my money on booze and women." He sounded a little disappointed.

After several minutes of polite conversation he and Keats rose and said goodbye. Just before they reached the door they heard a clear, tiny voice coming from behind the desk. They turned around slowly. The six-foot-six virologist was standing there holding the sugar-cube-sized tape recorder between his thumb and forefinger.

"It's Hideo Takayama's acceptance speech in Stockholm," he exclaimed apologetically. "He won the Nobel Prize in Medicine this year."

That night Annie Laurie served Keats his favorite dish, porterhouse steak with a baked potato. He had brought home a cold bottle of Sangria, first because he liked it and second because it cost only a dollar eighty-nine. He drank most of it himself. After dinner they sat in the living room looking through the papers to see if anything of interest was on television. They could find nothing. It was then that he decided to bring her up to date on the news of the virus killer even though he knew that he would soon regret his weakness. Any unpleasantness he could always blame on the Sangria. As an introduction he explained how he had cured Charlie Prince. Her years at the record room enabled her to understand the scientific terminology. Finally he gave her a complete account of the performance of Professor Choate's mad technician. He was careful not to reveal that he had returned half of the priceless solution to the Medical Center.

"So you still have six doses left," she said.

He kept silent. He knew that if he had told her the reason why he had only three left, she would have become very angry.

"It may be fifty years before anybody discovers the formula for a virus killer," she continued. "After your supply is used up there may be nothing like it for generations. You've got a gold mine. What are you going to do with it?" When he did not answer her, she said in despair, "You're like a member of a religious order who has taken a vow of poverty. Only you have a wife. You're fifty-four. Your practice is slipping away. You're on the skids. Who is going to take care of me in my old age?"

He shook his head. "I don't know, I don't know!"

He picked up a medical journal, walked into his bedroom, and closed the door. Although that month's issue was devoted to virology, he found himself unable to read a page. He lay down on his bed and stared at the ceiling.

8

LATE THE following Saturday afternoon Annie Laurie Keats climbed up the subway steps with nothing to show for her day's shopping but sore feet. Almost every Saturday morning she went downtown to buy clothes and shoes. Almost every Saturday afternoon she returned empty-handed. The dresses were either too short or too long, too cheap or too expensive, too fancy or too simple. And shoes which would make her comfortable had not yet been devised. Since the empty taxis all displayed off-duty signs, she decided to walk the six blocks home. On her left was Adams: off to her right the thirty-five-story apartment building in which Tunbridge Wells lived. The girls in the record room had often told her about his remarkable bedroom. The ceiling and walls were said to consist of cunningly joined mirrors placed there so that both partners in the sexual act could see exactly what was going on in any position they chose to assume. The centerpiece was a huge circular bed covered with a coal-black, stain-resistant spread. Sexual intercourse was never performed between the sheets, only on top of the black spread, which presumably revealed the Rubens, Titian, and even El Greco flesh tones of the women to the greatest advantage. The typist in charge of the nursery records, a beautiful Negress, said that she understood why he never had taken a black girl to bed. He would have had to go out and buy an expensive stain-resistant white cover just for the night. One of the older stenographers added that the dozens of mirrors must have made the room look like a Naples whorehouse when the fleet was in.

Some men are born whoremasters. Some have whoremastery thrust upon them, by women, of course. Wells belonged in both categories. He had devised a motor which at the touch of one of two buttons caused the bed to revolve slowly, almost imperceptibly, either clockwise or counterclockwise according to his whim. In complete control of himself and his partner during the sexual act, he managed to prolong the performance to inordinate lengths. More than one woman was known to have said in delighted amazement, "Do you realize that we made six revolutions before we reached a climax!" Naturally, he was not always at his best. On those occasions a touch of another button enabled him to increase the tempo of the bed while he was in the middle of coitus so that he could preserve his reputation as a six-circuit man. It was like speeding up a turntable from thirty-three to seventy-eight rotations a minute while the record was playing. Part of his success was due to his amazing ability to choose only women he was able to satisfy. In his lexicon of sexuality there was no such word as "frigid." His partners in turn considered him the greatest revolutionist since Lenin. They loved the merry-go-round that lived up to its name.

Annie Laurie Keats believed only half of what she had heard about Wells. Still, that half sounded a thousand times more attractive than anything that she could say about her husband. She could not help feel that Jim had married her under false pretenses. A Park Avenue doctor who proposed to a woman guaranteed, at least by implication, that he could support a wife. Of what use was a marriage which forced her to do not only all the work at home but hold down a full-time job as well? Annie Laurie felt that in contrast to his treatment of her, she had been honest with him. In the early weeks of their relationship she had told him that she could not have children because pelvic inflammatory disease had sealed off her tubes. After their marriage she had submitted to repeated attempts by a gynecologist to blow them open. She had allowed him to do everything, she often said, but hitch her vagina to the tire-inflating machine at the Mobil gas station around the corner. Was it her fault that nothing worked? She was guilty only of marrying a loser. She had been a beauty once. She could have gone all the way, maybe even latched on to someone like Tunbridge Wells. He was certainly going all the way. Unfortunately, he had not been at Adams when she was young.

As she walked up Lexington Avenue she recalled the biggest

triumph of her marriage. Three years before, she had stopped Jim from going to bed with her once and for all. In the old days it had been three times a week, as regular as clockwork. He would say, "Would you like to make love?" in the same tone of voice he would have used if he were asking her to go to the movies. It was not as bad as the "Let's have a party" one of her early lovers would whisper when he got the urge, but it was bad enough. After their marriage there had never been anything spontaneous about Jim's lovemaking. He would never slip his hand down her dress or take her clothes off as she sat on the couch. He hadn't pulled down a zipper in eight years. No, it was always the same routine. He would go into the toilet and take off his clothes. She was supposed to strip outside. Next he would gargle with Lavoris; that was a romantic sound for you, just the thing to put a woman in the mood! Then he would splash Canoe on his face, and, after a moment's hesitation, rub a little above his penis. That was supposed to make him more attractive. She would never forget the smell of Lavoris and Canoe. The combination was enough to make a woman throw up. Then the main event would begin. They would flop into bed as naked as two plucked chickens. He would play with her breasts, first the right, then the left. After a few minutes of this he would pull on her nipples, first the right, then the left. Never the other way around. That would have broken the routine. Next he would suck her nipples, a two-hundred-forty-pound infant at her breast. That always took a long time. Maybe he thought there was milk there. Then he would begin to move down, kissing her belly from north to south with a brief intermission while he inspected her navel. She could never figure out what he expected to find there. An Oriental dancing-girl's jewel, perhaps. Putting his lips to her pubic hair always excited him. She could tell from the way he breathed. At last he would spread her thighs and go to work down there. He called it cunnilingus, and it was supposed to give her a big thrill, like a trip to Paris. He could never say he was sucking her off, or doing a blow job. Oh, no, not he. He was the kind of man who couldn't call a cunt a cunt. Not in front of a woman. After this he would come back up and kiss her on the lips. That and the Lavoris and the Canoe. It was a miracle she didn't puke. But the grand finale was approaching. She had to spread her legs so that he could enter her body. Fair is fair, though. He had the biggest organ she had ever felt. And he was no in-and-out man. He really hung in there. The trouble was you'd think he had the ball on fourth down with one yard to go—up her vagina, unfortunately. When he came, the noise was unbelievable. He couldn't come quietly like a gentleman. Oh, no! You'd think a hydrogen bomb had gone off. Then he would roll off her and say, "Thank you." For what? For letting him masturbate into her vagina? He was the world's greatest sucker—next to her.

She decided to walk past the thirty-five-story phallic tower where Tunbridge Wells lived. After all, it was on her way home. She turned the corner and peered into the lobby. At that moment she felt a tap on her shoulder. She looked around and saw Wells, tall and thin, walking by her side. She thought of a saying she had heard as a little girl in Flushing: "Tall and thin gets further in, but short and thick is the better prick." She knew better now. When you'd felt one, you'd felt them all, she was convinced.

"You look flushed and tired," he said. "Is everything all right?"

"Everything except my feet and my disposition."

"Come up to my place for a minute. It's this house right here. I've got some wonderful foot-ease I can spray on your feet. Through your stockings," he added hastily when he saw her face tighten. "And I'll give you a cold drink, anything from milk to absinthe."

As they walked through the lobby the building superintendent, concealed by the shadows, watched them carefully. Another Wells Saturday afternoon special, he said to himself. They all had the same brand on the fourth finger of the left hand. Obviously Saturday afternoon was the best time for a busy pediatrician and a positive necessity for a working woman. Wives, whether they had a job or not, would find it hard to break away from their husbands at night without being caught or at least arousing suspicion. The moment the elevator door opened and the light flashed on Annie Laurie's face, he recognized her. He was shocked. Keats had introduced her to him years ago when he had brought his boy to the office for a routine check-up. She and her husband were about to go on their vacation. This was one hell of a way, he reflected, to treat a fine man like the doctor.

When Annie Laurie crossed the threshold of the apartment, she thought of a song from one of Noel Coward's albums, "A Room with a View." This one was on the thirty-second floor, and she was willing to bet that on a clear day you could see Maxim's. It was furnished with disarming simplicity, and every piece was good. She thought of her own furniture, which had long been ready for the Salvation Army.

"Sit in the corner of that big couch," said Wells as he walked toward another room. "It's the most comfortable place in the house." He returned with a spray can. "Take off your shoes. You'll get instant relief."

He was right. In a moment her feet felt cool and comfortable.

"What will you have?" he asked her as he put the spray can on a small bar at the other end of the room. "I've sometimes wondered what would happen if I squirted a little of this foot-ease into the drinks. Maybe it would become soul-ease and make the world look good."

"A tall scotch and soda with lots of ice, please."

"That makes two," he said.

He returned with the drinks, handed her one, and sat down on a chair near the couch. She noticed that he had made them with Chivas Regal.

"My husband really doesn't have a chance of getting that thirty-five-thousand-dollar-a-year director's job, does he?" she asked suddenly.

Wells looked down and swirled the ice in his glass. "He will be very seriously considered," he answered slowly. "He should be very seriously considered. But unfortunately he is getting on in years, not only chronologically but in his attitudes as well. He must be twenty years older than you."

"Sixteen."

"That makes you my age." He frowned. "It also makes your husband part of a different generation. In his day the big words were work, loyalty, discipline, and devotion. So what happened? This generation is saddled with crime, pollution, war, and inflation. The young are not impressed with old virtues which failed to keep us out of the mess we are in. Blood, sweat, and tears have become a rock-and-roll group. Churchill's triad has been replaced by education, communication, and participation. At least the residents think so. The trouble with your husband, great clinician though he may be, is that he has never tried to establish a rapport with the house staff. He still doesn't realize that in 1973 a resident is a doctor whose time has come."

"He believes in population control, starting with the population of residents at Adams. He thinks it should be cut in half so that each of them will learn what it's like to do a day's work."

"You see! He still can't get it through his head that residents are a hospital's immortality, its sperm, so to speak."

"He would agree to that. He thinks the house staff is screwing the hospital."

Wells laughed. "I wish he would think of it more as a love affair. I wish he would stop antagonizing so many people at Adams. You ought to tell him that more flies are caught with honey than with vinegar." He paused. "I can't answer your question completely. I don't know who the next director of Pediatrics will be. But I will say this. Coins, stamps, wine, and letters by famous men become more valuable with age. Hospital doctors do not."

"I'm sorrier for me than for him. I could use the money. Holding down a full-time job on top of being cook, housekeeper, and laundress at home is not my idea of how a doctor's wife should spend her life."

"Maybe you won't have to. A few days ago your husband saved the life of a boy everyone thought would die."

"Yes, I know."

"My chief, Dr. Dummer, told me that he used a substance called interferon. But I'm sure there's more to it than that. Do you know what he's playing around with?"

"Yes, an unknown substance, a virus killer."

"He's not putting you on, is he? Do you know where he keeps it and how much he has?"

"Yes."

"Then you're in. Throw out the mink, bring home the sable. All you have to do is persuade him to have the stuff analyzed. Once he has the formula, he can easily take out a patent. Since he is an ethical doctor, he should set up a charitable foundation and give it the patent and the formula absolutely free of charge. The foundation in turn will distribute the formula to all the pharmaceutical companies in the country with instructions to mass produce it at a reasonable profit for the benefit of mankind. All the foundation will ask for itself is ten percent of the product's gross sales so that it can improve and eventually perfect the new drug. In the Old Testament it states that a man must give one tenth of his earnings to charity. You expect the drug companies to cough up the biblical tithe. Have you any idea how much business they do? Eli Lilly alone grosses almost a billion dollars a year. Of course, a research foundation needs a director. What better man could be found than the discoverer of the new miracle medicine, Dr. James Keats? An iron-bound contract with the foundation he himself has established will be drawn up guaranteeing him one hundred thousand dollars a year until he is seventy. There will be a cost-of-living escalator clause. He can't come out of this deal with less than a million and a half, conveniently divided up into sixteen installments for tax purposes. You'll be able to quit your job. And you'll have the world in the palm of your hand."

"You don't know my husband."

"Evidently not. But there's more than one way to skin a cat. Especially if you don't forget where the magic medicine is hidden."

He stood up, sat down next to her on the couch, and took her glass. "Another drink? Freshen it up?"

"No, thank you." She knew the technique from the old days before she had met Jim.

He put his arm around her waist and held it there. Then he raised his hand slowly until he had her breast. Jeez, he said to himself, it's as tense as a toy balloon, only small and heavy, a regular Venus de Milo boobie. He watched her face. She was staring straight ahead with the blind gaze of a statue by Phidias. Didn't they paint the eyes in those days? They would have had to use a bright blue Tyrian dye for this one. He reached across her chest with his other hand and pulled the zipper in the front of her dress down to her brassiere. She smiled. She had forgotten what it was like to have a man undress her. She seemed to remember now that the last time it had happened she was wearing buttons. Wells smiled, too. There was life in the statue after all. It was a little out of his line but he wouldn't mind playing Pygmalion to her Galatea. Besides, any man who turned down a chance to lay a beautiful woman like this should have his penis examined. Very carefully he pulled down the zipper another inch. She bent over, put on her shoes, and walked to the table where her handbag lay. He noticed that she had not even bothered to zip up her dress.

"You're still in love with your husband, aren't you?" he asked, looking up at her from the couch.

"No," she answered coldly, "I'm menstruating."

Just before she closed the door she pulled up her zipper and said, "Thank you for the drink and the foot-ease."

He sat motionless on the couch for a few minutes. What a bitch, he said to himself. Everything so proper, proper. He was willing to wager that when she was young she had told each of her lovers that she had lost her virginity playing squat tag in an asparagus patch. Still, he would have liked to get her into bed, just to see what she would do. He had never tried a cold one before.

Annie Laurie hurried along Lexington Avenue on painless feet. He was certainly attractive, she said to herself, but she would be damned if she was going to crawl into bed with him unless she got something in return. What she liked most about him, even more than his good looks, was his business ability. He had a perfectly practical scheme for ethically getting a million and a half dollars for a drug which Jim was going to give away for nothing. Maybe she and Wells could work out something together. When she got home Jim was in the living room reading the *New York Times*. She tried hard to be pleasant and found herself chatty once again. After she had brought in the drinks, she said,

"I worry about your virus killer. Do you still keep it in that unlocked refrigerator at Adams?"

He nodded.

"Aren't you afraid someone will steal it?"

"Why would anybody steal it? Nobody at the hospital would have the guts to inject it intravenously."

Wells had dinner at a French restaurant in his building and then went to see the *Last Tango in Paris,* which he had missed the first time around. Brando certainly didn't know how to handle women, he decided. No wonder he ended up with a bullet in his belly. He returned home at eleven and undressed immediately. The virus killer was on his mind. Already he had forgotten his fanciful scheme for making a million and a half dollars, just as he always put from his mind the moment he uttered them the extravagant promises he made to friends and acquaintances alike. He could never resist the temptation to play the role of the man of influence, the big shot who could get things done. Tonight, however, he was less interested in commercially exploiting the virus killer for others than in getting his hands on it for himself. If he could use it on the child of a trustee, it would certainly give him an advantage in the contest for the directorship of Pediatrics, probably a decisive advantage. You never could have too many guns on your side. He would have to work through Annie Laurie. He gave a wry smile. She was the only woman who had ever walked out on him. Maybe he was slipping.

He put on a pair of black Sulka pajamas and lay down on the circular bed. Immediately it picked up speed and, whirling like a top, threw him to the floor. By the time he got to his feet it was motionless. He examined the button. It was in the off position. Again he lay down on the bed. This time it revolved even faster than before, dumping him a second time. Jeez, he said to himself, even the damn bed was rejecting him. He pulled out the plug, turned off the light, threw off the cover, and got in between the sheets. It took him a long time to fall asleep. He dreamed of Annie Laurie in a bubble bath. Suddenly the heavens were filled with toy balloons, exact replicas of what he imagined her breasts were like. He ran after them, vainly trying to clutch one while a thirty-five-piece swing band played "I'm Always Chasing Rainbows." Very appropriate, he thought. Rainbows, the giant breasts of the skies! No nipples, though. Well, you couldn't have everything.

The first thing he did on Monday morning was to arrange to have the bed repaired. The second was to find out from a closemouthed woman in the record room the name and telephone number of the insurance company where Annie Laurie worked.

9

THE JOHN QUINCY ADAMS Hospital Medical Board met in the conference room promptly at four o'clock every Wednesday afternoon. It was made up of the directors of the seven major departments, surgery, medicine, obstetric-gynecology, pediatrics, anesthesiology, the laboratories, and X-ray. Not only was it responsible for the medical affairs of the hospital, it was supposed to represent the three hundred and fifty doctors who held subordinate positions on the staff. In a sense it did, the way a war-time general represented the army he commanded. Ultimate power, however, did not rest in its hands. Its decisions and appointments were subject to the approval of a self-perpetuating board of thirty trustees.

In the past, the trustees had been expected to make up the deficit and keep the room rates down. They had accomplished these tasks by means of generous contributions. Today, only antiquarians remembered their charitable exploits. In the modern world, skyrocketing costs had resulted in their playing a relatively minor role in the financing of the hospital. The private room which under Mr. Gulbanian's regime had cost fifteen dollars a day now went for two hundred; and the ward bed in which the patient had once slept for three dollars maximum now had a one-hundred-dollar price tag. In 1972 inflation, increased labor costs, residents', directors', and administrators' salaries, food, and the purchase and use of sophisticated equipment had brought the budget up to forty million dollars. To meet this the trustees contributed less than two hundred thousand. The rest had been obtained from patients and third parties, the city, the state, Medicare, Medicaid, Blue Cross, Major Medical, and other insurance companies. Even if the trustees had been twice as generous, their donations would have amounted to less than one percent of the cost of running the institution. They still gave of their leisure time, their experience, and their judgment. But not of their hard cash. And they were careful not to relinquish any of their power.

Meeting a deficit would have put too great a strain on their financial resources. Attacking the problems inherent in running a forty-million-dollar-a-year enterprise would have taken up too much of their lives. They sidestepped these responsibilities by hiring a corps of experts to deal with the day-by-day affairs at Adams. They were called administrators and their chief was I. M. Hexter. Previous generations would have termed him the superintendent. Today's hospitals had polished up the title to chief executive officer or even president. At Adams he was called, rather simply, the Administrator, and with a capital A. He had flat-topped hair over a closely shaven, no-nonsense face and dressed conservatively and well. He looked like a bank president, and in a sense that was what he was. A physicist who had unsuccessfully asked him for a job remarked that the temperature of his personality approached absolute zero. Jim Keats wondered how he had passed his premarital blood test. He was sure that no blood had ever flowed. Hexter was cold, calculating, and polite. Requests he usually referred to an assistant or a committee, knowing quite well that they would not be acted upon. And he made a point of never going out of his way to help anyone. Such attributes were far from handicaps in a hospital administrator.

Most people would have thought that he had been hired to see to it that the employees were efficient, the service smooth, the food first class, and the hospital clean. As a matter of fact Adams was no longer as spotless nor its food as good as in the old days. A large faction of the employees did a far from satisfactory job. And in some areas the service was shameful. Yet the trustees were not perturbed. They had hired Hexter not to improve the hospital but to make sure that it ran in the black.

In the past, one of the methods of measuring the standing of a hospital was to find out how deeply it operated in the red. Prestigious institutions had prestigious deficits. Their boards of trustees were in reality boards of philanthropists. The members of the board at Adams, on the contrary, wanted to be connected with a good hospital, cheap. Hexter simply had to keep his budget in the black. If he did not, he must have reasoned, where would the additional money come from? Certainly not from his trustees. Money did not buy what it used to. During the Depression a gift of two million dollars would have put up a building big enough to house a hundred patients. Today, it would run Adams for two and a half weeks. Voluntary hospitals were becoming too expensive for modern trustees. That was why administrators were necessary.

At Adams the trustees were more interested in signing edicts than checks. One such decree had just stated that starting October 1973 the administrator, who was a layman, would become part of the medical board. The doctors were outraged. Their deliberations, especially those about the character and ability of new appointees or candidates for promotion, had always been conducted in the strictest secrecy. They were appalled at having to accept a weekly breach in security. Finally, a compromise was reached. Henceforward, the administrator would sit with the seven-man medical board, but without a vote. The directors agreed that if they were forced to have the trustees' spy among them, it was important to make certain that he could not cast a decisive ballot.

At exactly four P.M. October twenty-fourth, Courtney Akt, Director of the Department of Obstetrics-Gynecology and president of the medical board, called the meeting to order. Although he had never been closer to China than Los Angeles, and although his ancestors came from Austria, he had a mandarin moon-face, kept tan by the summer's sun and the winter's sun lamp, which women found mysteriously attractive. And by the nature of his specialty all his patients were women. Then there was the tough, Sinatralike speaking voice. But these were not the attributes which had made him such a success. His large and fashionable practice he owed to his brother, one of the all-time great Hollywood directors. This powerful and persuasive man had sent him a seemingly unending stream of famous cinema actresses ever since he had opened his office. By now there was hardly a rich woman with a pelvic disorder left in New York who had not succumbed to the temptation of consulting the gynecologist who had operated upon so many Hollywood stars and starlets. Unfortunately, his brother had not been able to supply him with much surgical ability. His lack of it could not be blamed solely on his skimpy training. It has often been said that men are born great surgeons. If that is so, Courtney Akt must have been born a poor one. One of the truly fine surgeons at Adams, a member of the Department of Surgery, not of the Department of Gynecology, said that he hacked his way through the female pelvis like a native with a machete making a path through the jungle. When the operative specimen, its anatomical lines obscured by the unskillful removal, arrived in the laboratory, the pathologist would give it a glance and without bothering to read the doctor's name on the label, sigh, "Courtney is at it again." His deficiencies did not deter him from performing large numbers of hysterectomies indiscriminately. More than one member of his staff, envious perhaps of his lucrative practice, had remarked that it was a wonder that a single adult uterus remained in New York. In spite of his inadequacies he continued to flourish. After all, he had unusual shrewdness, an authoritative manner, a face which evoked glimpses of the mysterious Orient, a tough-guy husky voice, and a devoted brother.

He looked up and down the long table in the conference room, counting his colleagues. "In the name of the medical board I want to welcome Mr. Hexter, our newest member."

Hexter decided to show a bit of warmth and modesty. "You all realize that I am in a precarious position. I have to walk the tightrope between the trustees on the one side and the doctors on the other. I expect to fall on my face."

"If you do," said John Scotti, Director of Medicine, "don't expect us to give you a big funeral."

Courtney Akt tapped on the table with his ballpoint pen but said nothing. Scotti was too tough and too powerful to tangle with just now. Almost half the beds in the hospital were occupied by patients on the medical service. The only other member of the board Akt expected he would have trouble with was Frank Ray, Director of the Department of Radiology. And Ray would be dead in six months. The gynecologist asked Grant to present the minutes of the last meeting. The Director of Laboratories opened a manila folder and read the routine report as if he were announcing a cure for cancer. For him this was the climax of the meeting. Bored but resigned, his colleagues did not interrupt him. When he finished, there was no discussion. The doctors feared that comments might endow the trivia they had just been forced to listen to with a spurious importance which would encourage him to make subsequent minutes even longer and more detailed. Grant was an emphasizer of the unimportant. If he had been asked to be the substitute speaker for Lincoln at Gettysburg, he would have delivered a lengthy report about the weather.

"All those in favor of accepting the minutes as presented, please say aye," said Akt.

For a moment Grant looked a little like a prime minister up for a vote of confidence. A few mumbled ayes put him at his ease.

"As most of you know," said the president of the medical board, "Evan Dummer reaches sixty-five, the mandatory retirement age, in December." He glanced at his six colleagues seated around the long table. All in their early or mid fifties, they were safe for at least ten years. All except Frank Ray. "If there are no objections, I will ask Grant to prepare a resolution expressing our thanks to Evan for what he has done for the hospital and our regret that he must leave."

Scotti grinned sardonically. "Don't make it too strong and I'll sign."

Clearly irritated, Akt rustled the papers in front of him. "With the permission of the medical board, I will have a notice posted tomorrow announcing that applicants for the position of director of Pediatrics will be accepted."

A few doctors nodded.

"According to the by-laws," Akt continued, "I must appoint a search committee to screen the candidates and recommend the two or three that are most suitable. My choices for the committee are Grant, Bligh, and Scotti with Bligh as chairman."

"I am sure the trustees would think it important," said Hexter, "for us to attract a large number of applicants for this position. A big list would enhance the prestige of the Department of Pediatrics and of the hospital."

Frank Ray, Director of Radiology, stirred uneasily. He was a politician of the Abe Lincoln type. Under his armamentarium of stratagems, surprises, traps, and blitzes lay his greatest weapon—his integrity. The coughing had begun three months before. Occasionally his sputum had been blood-tinged. Seated in his little office, surrounded by his huge X-ray machines, he had refused at first to have a chest plate taken. When he agreed at last, the film had shown an inoperable cancer of the lung. The tumor had probably been inoperable from the start. Bronchoscopy had only confirmed the diagnosis. His devoted staff would not let him see his plates, quoting the old maxim that a doctor who treats himself has a fool for a patient. The faked typewritten report which was handed to him stated that he had a localized bronchitis of the right lower lobe with early bronchiectasis. He was not deceived, especially when he learned that he was to receive cobalt therapy in his own department. But he pretended that he was. He felt it would be churlish to disappoint so many concerned people. He knew that within a year there would be a new director of Radiology. Members of the medical board were probably already making secret overtures to prominent radiologists. Never mind if I'm the last to know that Adams is unfaithful to me, he said to himself. I would not be the first doctor to be cuckolded by a hospital.

"I think it is cruel," he said, "to falsely arouse the hopes of the pediatricians here at Adams, young and old, and a dozen or two unwanted ones in other hospitals by enticing them to apply for this position when all the while we know that we are going to give it to either Keats or Wells. How many times in this very room have we interviewed thirty doctors for one position and sent at least a third of them home each under the delusion that the job was his, whereas the winner had in fact been unofficially chosen before the notice went up! I can see each of the poor bastards telling his wife as soon as he got home which remark by which director had finally convinced him that he was number one. I'm going to sit this one out."

Scotti put his arm around Ray's shoulders. "You're right, Frank, but try to look at it from the trustees' point of view. To them, two applications mean that nobody really wants the job, thirty that it's very valuable. And they want their bauble, Adams, to be very valuable."

"All right, we'll have thirty de jure candidates in keeping with the laws of the trustees and two de facto candidates in keeping with the laws of reality."

"There is another possibility," said Airov, Director of Anesthesiology. "We could seriously consider the appointment of an outsider, a big name."

William Bligh, Director of Surgery, snorted. Cold of heart and sadistic, he reminded so many people of Charles Laughton in *Mutiny on the Bounty* that he was commonly referred to as Captain Bligh. A bachelor of fifty-six, he had become a millionaire by inheriting large sums of money from rich relatives who were considerate enough to die with remarkable regularity every few years. His stinginess was proverbial. No one had ever known him to perform a generous act.

When accused of selfishness, he would reply that he had never signed a contract to be munificent. He had no dependents. He changed his chauffeur and servants frequently, not because they were unsatisfactory but because he did not want them to become old retainers who might naively imagine that he would provide them with a pension. Toward himself he was magnanimous. His living quarters, clothes, cars, food, amusements, and vacations were the finest. He had no hobbies. He lived for himself and surgery, in that order. People meant little to him; operations everything. When he performed a successful one he was heartless about the bill. But since he had never had a money worry in his life, he was unfamiliar with the anguish of poverty. When he had entered Adams as an intern thirty-two years before, his father had given him an automobile. What made the gift so unusual was that a chauffeur came with it. Bligh never bothered to learn to drive. There would always be someone to do it for him, he reasoned. In the last year of his residency, he once left the hospital without any of the fine cambric handkerchiefs his father used to regularly send him on Christmas. Dropping in at Woolworth's, he discovered that a handkerchief could be bought for a nickel, considerably less than the cost of having one of his own hand laundered. Thereafter he bought all his handkerchiefs at the five-and-ten, and threw them away after using them once, an economy of which he was inordinately proud. At the hospital he was commonly referred to as a prick until someone remarked that it was improper to so demean a noble organ.

When he was fifty-five he first noticed a tremor of his right hand. His left was comparatively steady. After this he used his shaky side as little as possible, especially when he was being observed. A cocktail, a cup of coffee, or a glass of water, especially if they were full, he would now invariably lift with his left hand. And he was careful never to pour a liquid from one vessel to another with his right. When he had to use it to manipulate an instrument during the examination of a patient in his office, he learned to rest a finger against an adjacent portion of the body to mask his tremor. His handwriting deteriorated but he wrote few prescriptions. Besides, a doctor's handwriting was supposed to be illegible. Before long he was permitting his residents to perform all the operations on his private and semiprivate patients although he remained on the other side of the table to give instructions. He believed that the members of the house staff would interpret this largesse as a sign of his interest in the young. On the contrary, they were well aware of the reason for his generosity. Toward his attendings, some of whom were as old as he, he acted more and more the bully. It was as if he were saying to each of them, "Yes, I admit that my right hand is unsteady, but before I get through with you, you will be trembling over your entire body." Two weeks before the meeting of the medical board, he noticed that his left hand was beginning to shake.

"Big names are no longer in private practice," he said. "They work full time in university hospitals. You're in for a shock, Leonid. You'll soon find out that the professors are not going to leave their research and their medical schools to work at Adams for thirty-five thousand a year. And to meet their financial demands would be a disgraceful extravagance."

Courtney Akt nodded. "And a good thing, too. The appointment of a single full timer to a clinical specialty here would open up the floodgates. We clinicians would be drowned. We would be replaced in no time by research professors who could not exercise their primary skills in this nonresearch hospital and who could not handle our case load since they had never had to earn a living by treating private patients."

"My guess," said Hexter, "is that the trustees would not be opposed to your bringing in an outsider if you should become deadlocked in choosing a successor to Dr. Dummer from among the members of his staff." He smiled. "But I think it is a little premature to talk of a full-time director at this time."

There was a deadly silence while each of the doctors tried to interpret the phrase "at this time."

"I have a confession to make," said Dummer at last. "Three and a half years ago when the pediatric service had come upon bad times I went to Professor Locke at the Medical Center for help. I was particularly interested in getting a young man to assist me in turning the service around. He gave me Bridge Wells and enough residents every year to put the department on its feet. You all know what happened. Pediatrics at Adams is flourishing. We have more residents per square foot than any pediatric department in the city. But to get something I had to give something. I promised Locke that when my time came, Bridge Wells would get my job. The advantages to the department would be very great, an eventual affiliation with the Medical Center

112

and the medical school. Luckily, the story has a happy ending. After working closely with Bridge for over three years, I can tell you that he deserves to be the next director of Pediatrics."

"Nobody knows the candidates as well as Evan," said Grant.

Bligh nodded. "When it comes to his successor, Evan Dummer holds the most important vote in the room."

Frank Ray coughed and put his handkerchief to his lips. When he removed it, the doctors could see that it was bloodstained. No one made any comments.

"Dummer, you acted improperly," he said. "This position was not yours to give. The medical board is not committed by your promise to Locke."

"I know, I know," said Dummer. "But the future of the Department of Pediatrics was at stake. We had no residents. You don't seem to realize that there is a direct statistical relationship between the standing of a department of pediatrics and the number of residents it can obtain. The great children's centers have thirty or forty apiece; the third-rate pediatric services maybe two or three. Statistics don't lie."

"But conclusions drawn from them may be erroneous. There is a direct, statistically proved correlation between the population of storks in northern Europe and the birth rate. The more storks there are, the more infants are born. The fewer storks there are, the fewer infants are born. The conclusion that could be drawn from the statistics is that storks bring babies. But a sophisticated group like this knows that they are brought by Brother Akt. The residents at the Harvard Children's Center are a response to its excellence. The residents in your department are a mask for its deficiencies."

Courtney Akt tapped on the table with his pen. "We are not here to evaluate the Department of Pediatrics."

"Maybe not," said Scotti, "but it's time we took off the gloves. See for yourself. Walk through Dummer's department. Half the time you'll see more residents than medical pediatric patients. Together with obstetrics, pediatrics has the lowest census in the house. While the Department of Medicine is turning away patients with cardiac infarctions, bleeding gastric ulcers, cancers, and strokes because it has no place to put them, Dummer is talking to his residents beside empty beds. He doesn't need residents. He needs patients."

"Gentlemen," said Courtney Akt, "may I remind you that we came here to declare the position of director of Pediatrics open and to appoint a search committee. We've done this. Now we have a long agenda ahead of us."

Bligh looked up from a sheet of paper on which he had been doodling with his left hand. "I don't doubt these statements for a moment. Nevertheless I have something I wish to bring up," he said. "It has been brought to my attention that Dr. Keats, the once famous football player, indulged in some hanky-panky on the pediatric service last week. A twelve-year-old boy lay dying with the Guillain Barré Syndrome. He had complete paralysis of all four extremities and partial paralysis of the muscles of respiration. He had been intubated by Airov and was on the Bennett respirator. No one would have given a nickel for his chances of recovery. Then Keats walked in and injected something into the boy's vein. Three hours later the little fellow was running around as if he had never been sick. Dr. Airov, you passed the endotracheal tube. Are my facts correct?"

"I don't understand what you have against football players," interrupted Scotti. "I used to be one myself. As a matter of fact I once played right tackle for Columbia and opened up holes for Jim Keats."

"Weren't you a little light for a tackle?" asked Bligh coldly.

"Yes, but I was fast and mean."

"You still are," said Bligh.

"Gentlemen," put in Airov, "do you mind if I answer Dr. Bligh's question?" Nobody said anything. "Yes, Bill, your facts are correct."

"Not being burdened with a wife," Bligh continued, "sometimes has its advantages. I had plenty of time to look up the literature. There is no specific treatment for the Guillain Barré Syndrome. No such dramatic cure has ever been reported. Evan, what did Keats inject?"

"I have been told that it was a solution of interferon," replied Dummer.

"That's strange. Everything I have read states that in humans interferon is either ineffective or at best a weak viral antagonist. Has Keats published anything? A preliminary report, perhaps? Read a paper before a medical society? Why hasn't he presented his findings so that the profession can decide whether his claims are valid?"

"Evidently he is not making any claims," said Ray. He put another handkerchief to his lips.

"Let me ask you this question," Bligh continued, turning to Grant.

"You're not only in charge of the laboratory but you're chairman of the research committee as well. Has Dr. Keats ever discussed his work with you?"

"Never. All I hear are wisecracks and insults. He's the Don Rickles of the hospital," said Grant.

"Evan, you're his chief," said Bligh. "Do you know what he is up to?"

Dummer shook his head.

"He certainly has never obtained permission from the medical board for any work of this kind," Bligh continued. "The more I think things over, the more I detect the smell of charlatanism in the air. His pseudoscientific secret remedies could cost the hospital a lot of money someday. If anything ever goes wrong, Adams could be sued for malpractice."

Scotti laughed and looked at the president of the medical board. "Do you think we should reprimand him for saving the life of one of his patients?"

"I'm not worried about malpractice," said Ray. "Bligh is so rich he could pay for any law suit out of his own pocket. Adams would not be stuck for a cent."

"And so generous," said Scotti, "that he would then divide up his fortune among the few indigent patients he still has and retire to a monastery."

Akt tapped on the table with his ballpoint pen. "Gentlemen, please stop horsing around. We have a long agenda ahead of us, and I have to pick up my brother at Kennedy Airport in an hour and a half."

"Maybe you could persuade your brother to fix old Dummer up with a young starlet," said Scotti. "She would be a farewell present from the medical board. I'm sure we would all be willing to help lay him on and lift him off."

10

THE NEXT morning Wells telephoned Annie Laurie at the insurance company where she worked. His bed had just been repaired. "Forgive me for interrupting you while you're on the job, but I wonder whether you would have a drink with me at my place this Saturday afternoon."

The only answer he received was a prolonged silence.

He tried again. "Absolutely no monkeyshines. I'm obsessed with your husband's virus killer, that's all."

"I'll have a drink with you at the Barclay at five this afternoon," she said.

"We might be seen. Don't you think it's a little dangerous?"

"Not as dangerous as coming to your apartment."

"All right, fine, the Barclay at five."

A thirty-eight-year-old Doris Day virgin, he said to himself as he hung up. A leader of the resistance. He had never tried an unwilling one before. He must be getting soft in the head. At least it was better than getting soft in the penis.

She was twenty minutes late when she walked toward his table in the cocktail lounge. He could see that she was going to be a pain in the ass. A beautiful pain, though. They both had scotch and soda.

"Annie Laurie is a strange name," he said. "Do you mind if I call you Ann?"

"If you want to take my name away from me, go ahead. Nobody has ever tried before. Be the first."

Ah, he said to himself, a virgin in name only.

She sipped her drink. "I was very much impressed with your scheme. Imagine, a million and a half dollars! The only trouble is that Jim could never carry it through. He lacks a business sense. He's not a money man. The solution might be for you to approach him and explain your proposition in detail. You could become the junior partner. He would handle the scientific end, you the financial."

"I'd like to hear a little more about this virus killer first. Exactly what is it?"

"All right, you're entitled to know."

She told him everything about the virus killer.

Wells looked thoughtful. "It must have taken a lot of guts for your husband to have injected that stuff into his own veins." He sipped his drink. "I'm surprised that Professor Choate harbored a mad technician all these years. He's evidently not as good a judge of character as he is of viruses. You must know, of course, that he is one of this country's most eminent scientists. He almost won the Nobel Prize." He smiled. "Of course, there's always one of those in every medical school." He took another sip of his drink. "How much does your husband have left?"

"Six doses, twelve ml." She did not know that her husband had returned three of those doses, six ml., to Choate.

Wells gave her a hard look. "I see. That's not very much, is it? From what you told me before, I thought that there would be much more. The other day I put a hypothetical question to a top-flight biochemist who is a good friend of mine. I asked him how long it would take to analyze a complicated solution which had an almost unbelievable therapeutic effect. You see, I was really looking out for your interests. He said it might take years." He made it sound as if the bad news were really Annie Laurie's fault. "What you've just told me makes things worse. When we've used up the twelve ml., where could we get more? We might very well not have enough for the analysis."

She smiled bitterly. "That means there won't be any charitable foundation, right?"

"I'm afraid not," said Wells. He was never upset when a bit of boasting or an unfulfilled promise brought disappointment to a gullible friend. He had learned that nobody ever reproached him.

"And the million and a half dollars goes down the drain. Right?" she said.

"Yes, but there is something else we can do," he said reassuringly.

"Tunbridge is a strange name. Do you mind if I call you Bridge?"

"Everyone does."

"Bridge, do you know what you are? You're nine tenths hot air and one tenth charm."

He reddened.

"My German grandmother would have called you a *Luftmensch*," she continued. "That's a man who lives up in the air, a man whose mind turns out extravagant schemes while his tongue drips promises he can never fulfill. 'Luft' means 'air' in German. No wonder you live on the thirty-second floor. From what I hear there's only one time when you deliver the goods. Like an expert balloonist you are said to be able to take a woman up to the clouds and bring her back unharmed. I believe it, especially if your balloon is filled with your own hot air." She smiled. "It's a skill, I suppose, the world can't do without. Only don't expect me to be a passenger."

"Touché. But you haven't asked to hear my other scheme. It's more practical but much more dangerous."

"Go ahead. I'm tired. I ache all over after a day's work. Bathe me in your fantasies."

He took a gulp of his drink. "No matter what happens, your husband is not going to get the job. Four of the seven men on the medical board are implacably opposed to him." He raised his hand. "True, I may not get it either. They may call in someone from the outside. But your husband will never be the next director."

"All right, we'll forget him."

"On the other hand, I have a good chance of being chosen. Dr. Dummer is backing me. If in addition to all that's going for me I could get my hands on the virus killer, I think my appointment would be assured. If I could pull off six miracles in the next two months, with the appropriate publicity, of course, I'm positive that the board of trustees would put so much pressure on the medical board that I would be a shoo-in. And that medicine from the Medical Center would work wonders for my career and my practice, too. The key word is publicity. Your husband is trying to keep the virus killer a secret. I would proclaim it from the housetops."

"And what would you say it was?"

"The most concentrated solution of interferon yet prepared. A well-known chemist whom I've known since we were kids would back me up. I once did him a big favor. The fact that he lives in Hawaii is the icing on the cake. The medical board wouldn't be apt to subpoena him."

"What would happen to Jim?"

"Nothing. He would be just where he was before he got the so-called interferon from Professor Choate. Six children will be saved. What difference does it make whether he saves little Mary Smith or I save little Mary Jones? For Christ's sake, I'm not going to use it on convicted murderers. Kids are kids. The only difference is that I know how to exploit my triumphs and he doesn't know how to exploit his. He's really a dog in the manger. If he's not able to use the virus killer for his own advantage, why should he prevent me from using it for mine? The beauty of the scheme is that nobody gets hurt." He finished his drink. "Aren't you going to ask me how I plan to get the virus killer from your husband?"

"You're going to buy it from him."

"He would never sell. And he would be horrified at my lack of ethics."

"You're absolutely right. So how would you get it?"

"I don't intend to get it. You would get it for me."

"Why should I do that?"

"That's the only thing I can't figure out. Another drink?"

"No. I have to go home and cook."

"I suppose you would stand up, give me a dirty look, and hurry away if I offered you money."

"No, my feet hurt." She looked at the ice in her glass. "One afternoon as I was coming home from grade school long, long ago, I saw my favorite aunt being evicted because she couldn't pay the rent. It was raining, and the furniture I used to play on was out in the street. The year I started to work in the record room my mother went on relief. What could I do on the salary they paid me? My sister was one of the first candidates for Medicaid. And my poor grandfather, the nice one, died on a free ward at Bellevue. No, I wouldn't walk away if you offered me money." She smiled. "I'm not interested in the mink and sables you dangled in front of me last Saturday, *Luftmensch*. All I want is security in my old age, a little house, free and clear, so that when my turn comes I won't be evicted because I can't pay the rent."

He reached across the table and patted her hand. "Get me this virus killer, and if they make me director, I'll give you my first year's salary, thirty-five thousand dollars, free and clear. I'll pay the gift tax." He waved his hand in front of her as if to forestall any protest she might make against his excessive generosity. "I'll be on the payroll for twenty-seven years. Sixty-five is the retirement age at Adams.

My total take will be almost a million dollars. That's in addition to my income from private practice. I can afford to give you thirty-five, especially since my grandmother left me a sizable inheritance when I was twenty-one."

"Yes, you can."

"If you put the money in the savings bank, it will double in ten years. If you prefer to invest it, I know a whiz of a stockbroker—not some employee, but a member of the firm—who can more than double it in one year. Then, if you put it in the savings bank, you will have a hundred and fifty thousand dollars in ten years. That should give you some security."

"Suppose they don't make you director?"

"Then I'll treat you to a month's vacation in Europe, either with or without me."

She laughed. "I think I'll call you LM. That's short for *Luftmensch*. You'll be forty soon. Your days of freeloading on pushovers are coming to an end. Before long women will expect more from you than a roll in the hay. You must be wandering in the clouds if you think I am going to throw away everything I have for a twenty-eight-day guided tour of Portugal. Jim may not be much of a husband, but he pays for the rent, the food, the electricity, and the telephone. Suppose he learns of your scheme and throws me out? No, dear LM, if I hand the virus killer over to you, and it's a big 'if,' I expect a check for thirty-five thousand dollars on delivery. You get six miracles for less than six thousand dollars apiece. With your business genius to guide you, you ought to end up with a nice profit. One thing I'm sure of. Moses, Jesus, and Merlin combined never made as much money out of their miracles as you will make out of yours."

"Suppose the stuff is no good anymore," he said. "Suppose it has lost its potency."

"You haven't lost yours, I hope. It's a package deal. I come with it. You'll have to take a chance on the virus killer and me."

He scratched his head. "All right, it's a deal, a package deal."

"One more thing. This won't be any afternoon's balloon ride. We'll have to have a more permanent relationship. In fact we are going to be as thick as thieves. That's because we *are* thieves."

She stood up. "Now I have to go and earn that money." As she walked away from the table he shook his head and said to himself, "The Sing-Sing Venus!"

A half hour later, as she sat reading the *Post* in her living room, she looked up and said to her husband, "Last night I could hear you snoring through two closed doors. That usually means you have something on your mind. What's worrying you this time?"

"Nothing. Next Wednesday I'm going to a three-day convention of the American Academy of Pediatrics in Boston. It won't cost anything though. 'Chip' Levine and his wife are putting me up. We used to see a lot of them when he was at New York Hospital, remember? And the old car should make it. The only thing I'm concerned about is that I really can't afford to lose the three days' income from my practice."

"I worry about something, too, only I don't snore about it. Why don't you keep the virus killer in this refrigerator or the one in your office. It would be a lot safer that way."

She did not expect him to pay any attention to her. She hoped he would not. Her suggestion was merely a ploy to find out whether the medicine was still in his laboratory refrigerator at Adams.

"Because you'd knock it over when you took out the milk," he answered. "And the girl at my office isn't much better. Last week she broke a thirteen-dollar bottle of immune globulin. I wouldn't trust her with yesterday's paper. Besides, I've got a ferocious beast to guard that icebox. He's tougher than Fafnir, the Wagnerian dragon who watched over the golden treasure of the Rhine."

"You mean that dog you saved from distemper?"

He nodded.

"He would probably lead the burglar to the virus killer," she said, "and then lick his hand."

He smiled and returned to the *New York Times*. After a moment he looked up. "Maybe you're right. I'll be away for three days, and God only knows what that Nazi bastard, Tugend, might do in my absence. First thing tomorrow I'm going to get two small 'eye' bolts and put one on the refrigerator frame, the other on the door. Then I'll fasten them together with a good padlock. You'll have one key. I'll have the other. Okay? If you have to take out the virus killer in an emergency, it's clearly labeled 'Interferon.'"

She turned pale but did not dare to try to make him give up this scheme that would incriminate her.

The next morning she telephoned Wells during his office hours. "We've had a setback. I'd like to see you tomorrow."

"Great. Four o'clock at my place. Don't fret. We'll work it out together."

She felt more confident at once. It was the voice, not the words, she decided, which gave her courage.

Promptly at four the following afternoon she entered an elevator in Wells's tower building. The superintendent stood in the shadows as he did regularly at this time. Watching for Wells's Saturday afternoon specials had become a hobby with him. They were easy to identify, first by their promptness and second by the brash way in which they called out, "Thirty-second floor, please," to the operator as if they were visiting a maiden aunt, or Little Red Riding Hood instead of the wolf. He was surprised to see that Mrs. Keats had been recalled for a repeat performance. This honor could only mean, he was sure, that she was hotter than a two-dollar pistol. He waited three minutes and then took the freight elevator to the thirty-second floor.

Wells opened the door at once.

"We're shutting off the hot water at nine o'clock Monday morning," said the superintendent.

Wells nodded and closed the door. The superintendent was quick to notice that the doctor had neither asked why the hot water was being turned off nor when it would be restored. And he had closed the door almost as soon as he had checked its opening swing. What was more important was that the superintendent had seen Annie Laurie's handbag on an end table.

Wells walked back through the foyer and sat down opposite her. "He's turning off the hot water Monday morning."

"My condolences," she said, "but you can outwit him. All you have to do is ignore what I'm going to tell you. Then we will both be in hot water."

"It's something pleasant to look forward to, but I will never ignore anything you tell me."

"I might as well reveal the secret. Jim keeps the virus killer in his laboratory refrigerator at Adams. Everything was sailing along smoothly until I had to put my two cents in. Next Wednesday he's going to the pediatric convention in Boston for three days. I tried to show my concern about the safety of his magic medicine in order to find out whether it was still in the same old place. I succeeded all right. And I convinced him to be more careful. He put a padlock on his refrigerator yesterday. There are only two keys. He has one. I have the other. If the virus killer is gone when he returns next Saturday, he will know, naive as he is, that I am the only one who could have taken it."

"Do you have the key with you?"

"Of course not," she answered curtly.

"That's all right. Now stop fretting. He's handed us everything on a silver platter. As soon as he leaves, we will go to his laboratory at Adams together. You will open the refrigerator with your key, and hand me the virus killer. I will then pour it into a sterile bottle which I will carefully place in my little black bag. Next I will squirt exactly twelve ml. of a harmless physiological saline solution into the original bottle and put it back in the refrigerator in the same position it was when your husband went away. Finally, you will lock the refrigerator and we will both walk out. When he returns, I guarantee that he will never detect the substitution."

"What will he think when he injects the solution into a child and nothing happens?"

"It can't do the child the slightest harm. He'll think the virus killer has deteriorated; that it's lost its potency. Does it have a preservative?"

"Not that I know of."

"There you are. Maybe it really has lost its effectiveness. In that case I'll be out thirty-five thousand dollars."

"No, you won't. You're getting something else."

He smiled. "I know."

"Not that," she said impatiently. "You're buying insurance. If the virus killer has held up this long, the chances are that it will hold up at least a couple of more months. You're insuring that Jim will not have the use of his magic medicine. Suppose you let him keep it and he performs six miracles. If that happens, don't you think that the trustees might see to it that he performs a seventh, that he becomes the next director?"

"All right, all right, I'm not complaining."

"Besides, the whole thing was your idea. Could I have a drink?"

He went to the bar and returned with two scotch and sodas.

"The only thing that disturbs me is the crummy way I am treating Jim," she said at last. "I can imagine how he is going to feel when he injects those kids and nothing happens. I'm really as bad as a marshal's wife who would creep out of bed in the middle of the night to substitute blanks for the bullets in her husband's Colt knowing that the next day he was going up against the most dangerous gunfighter in Dodge City."

"Oh, stop fretting, Ann. No one is going to get hurt. Your husband didn't discover the virus killer the way Fleming discovered penicillin. He just got hold of it by dumb luck. Six children will be saved. What difference does it make whether he saves them or I do?"

He stood up and sat down next to her on the couch. "I don't know any other way to stop you from fretting."

He undressed her slowly and methodically while he kissed her. She was tense, wondering whether she would respond to him. Still this was better than the gargling, the Lavoris, and the Canoe. When her clothes were off he lifted her up and carried her into the bedroom. The mirrors repeated what she already knew—that a fully dressed man was walking around with a naked woman in his arms. She wondered who kept all those mirrors so clean, especially the ones on the ceiling. He did not seem tired while he was carrying her nor relieved when he was able to lay her down on the bed, probably, she reflected, because he had had so much practice transporting women into the bedroom in this manner. He undressed slowly and gravely, hanging his carefully folded clothes on a chair close to her. The suit, she noticed, came from Dunhill's made-to-order department. It must have cost at least four hundred dollars. Jim got his suits at Rothman's during sales for fifty-nine fifty. The label on the shirt said Sulka. Jim shopped at Gimbel's basement. He was such a cheapskate about clothes. Here everything was elegant and expensive. The black spread she was lying on was soft and luxurious. She was not concerned about pleasing Wells. Men would get into bed with anyone who had two breasts and a vagina. They weren't picky. They didn't demand two breasts and two vaginas even though such an abnormality would undoubtedly have doubled their pleasure. No, they were easy to please. She was worried about her own reactions. That Wells might not be able to satisfy her was her only fear. And not because she craved sexual release. Only because she wanted to be reassured that she was a normal woman.

He lay down quietly next to her. Springs did not creak as they used to when her two-hundred-forty-pound husband landed on her single bed at home. After she felt a few reasonable caresses, she closed her eyes so that she would not have to see her body being fondled on the ceiling. Wells took a strand of her hair and kissed it. With his other hand he pressed the "counterclockwise" button. Immediately the bed began to whirl, tossing them both violently to the floor.

He knelt beside her. "Are you hurt?"

"Of course not," she answered as she sat up. "Do you think I'm a fairy princess who can feel a pea through twenty mattresses? I was brought up in a tough neighborhood. Girls threw rocks at each other. Are you hurt?"

"Only my pride."

He helped her to her feet. She felt less tense, relieved in fact. Even a highly sexed woman could not be expected to respond to a man after something like this, she knew. While she was in the bathroom rubbing her buttocks with a towel, he pressed the "off" button on the bed and watched it for a moment to see that it remained in place.

"What a way to seduce a woman!" she said as she entered the room. "Do you take out Blue Cross, Blue Shield, and Major Medical for your conquests?"

He smiled ruefully. The counterclockwise motor had evidently gone out of control in spite of the fact that he had just had the entire mechanism overhauled. Everything depended now on whether the clockwise motor was working properly. They lay down on the bed together. Again she closed her eyes so that she would not have to see what was happening on the ceiling. Again she felt him take a strand of her hair.

"Please!" she said, disengaging it with a smile. "The last time you did that I landed on the floor."

He pressed the "clockwise" button. Slowly and smoothly the bed began to revolve. She sighed, bent her knees, and spread her thighs. Very adroitly he penetrated her body. She was certainly well lubricated, he noted with approval. Some of the old bags he had had in this bed were as dry as death. She smiled. There was going to be no cunnilingus, she realized, and her heart lifted. Jim must have some French blood in him, she decided. As soon as he got into bed, he acted like a foreigner. There would be none of that this afternoon, Annie Laurie was glad to see. The man on top of her was a straight up-and-down American, thank God.

"I hope what happened just now," he said without interrupting the rhythm, "didn't get us off to a bad start."

She took his head between her hands and gently pushed it away so that she could see him. "Are you really New York's finest lover? Is this the face that launched a thousand hips?" She pulled back her hands suddenly. "Then why the hell do you have a cockamamie bed that throws people on the floor!" Then she laughed.

"Ann, you're not supposed to laugh while you're making love. The sexual act isn't funny."

"Henry Miller thinks it is," she said.

"You're not in bed with Henry Miller."

"I'm glad."

The bed turned around and around endlessly. The up-and-down motion never ceased. It was all so nice, she felt, like having one's back rubbed or being on the verge of a sneeze. She had heard that the bed often made six revolutions before the lovers' needs were satisfied. Surely this afternoon it must have made six hundred. At long last she knew the itch of desire. Suddenly she felt his orgasm inside her. He did it like a gentleman. A wolf he of course was, but he didn't huff and puff and blow the house down like Jim. Seconds later she had an orgasm, too, a ladylike one that was quite satisfying, she thought.

He rolled off her body. After a moment he sat up and looked down at her. "Excuse the indelicacy, Ann," he said, "but you're built like a brick shit house."

She smiled and opened her eyes. "You're not exactly a hunchback of Notre Dame yourself."

They lay still for a few minutes. Then she sat up and said,

"I have to go home and cook."

She flung on her clothes rapidly, putting on her stockings inside out. As soon as they walked into the living room he said,

"Sit down, Ann, please, just for a minute. We have to plan. We're not going to be Watergate plumbers. We're going to be gifted amateurs. I suggest Wednesday night for the job. Then, if something goes wrong, we can try again Thursday and Friday. I want you to walk into the main lobby at Adams at exactly nine o'clock Wednesday night. And don't forget to bring the key. You will be visiting a patient or going to the ladies' room or checking on your husband's lab if anyone spots you. Promptly at nine I will walk through the lobby wearing my long white coat and carrying my black bag. In it will be my burglar tools, syringes, cotton, alcohol, a one-hundred-ml. bottle of physiological saline solution, and an empty, sterile bottle for the virus killer. We'll nod to each other and walk into the elevator separately. And we'll get out at the seventh floor separately. Nobody is ever in the research laboratories at night. If, however, fate is unkind and we are seen there together, you, the proud wife, are showing me your husband's lab and the distemper dog whose life he saved. It's not as if the two of us were caught in a motel."

She stood up. "I'll be there. And don't forget to bring a certified check for thirty-five thousand dollars. Cash would be cumbersome."

The superintendent was standing in the shadows as she walked through the main lobby. He liked to see them when they came out. He noticed that she was no longer wearing her brassiere.

11

THE FOLLOWING Monday morning Keats's secretary-receptionist walked into the consultation room and said,

"Mr. Roach, the super of that fancy apartment house near Adams, is here without an appointment and without his son."

"Bring him in," said Keats. "We're not busy."

As soon as the man sat down Keats asked, "Where's your boy?"

"I didn't come here to consult you, Doctor," said the superintendent. "I came to warn you."

During the three years that Keats had been Columbia's varsity fullback, the assistant coaches had often warned him against outstanding players on opposing teams. After his sophomore season he decided that he functioned best when he simply followed his blockers, ran for daylight, or dragged a tackler for those extra four yards.

Since then he had never been upset by warnings. He said nothing now.

"You'll have to excuse me if I'm a little garrulous," said Roach. "Ever since my wife died I talk too much. But then I never got a word in edgewise while she was alive." He smiled. Keats did not smile back.

"In the old days," continued the super, "the king used to have the bearer of bad tidings executed. If his majesty couldn't destroy the news, he could at least destroy the messenger. I know this, but I came here anyway." He hesitated. "There's a stud in my building, a high-class fucker."

"What has this got to do with me?" asked Keats.

"It has everything to do with you, Doctor," answered Roach. "He's young, rich, and handsome. You're not." He raised his hand. "I don't mean to be disrespectful. I'm just telling the truth. On the other hand, he's a prick, literally and in spades, while you are a fine man."

Such praise would not lead to a Nobel Prize, Keats knew, but it was better than a malpractice suit.

"Almost every Saturday afternoon at four o'clock a different woman goes up to his apartment," Roach went on. "They are all expensively dressed, over thirty-five, fairly attractive, and married. Once in a blue moon somebody is called back for an encore. This bastard can pick and choose. Broads like these would never have anything to do with me, even if I paid for it. You're wondering how I know that they all go to his apartment, aren't you?" he asked, even though he could see that Keats was not showing the slightest curiosity. "First they all call out 'thirty-second floor' in a loud voice, as if they were going to Bergdorf Goodman and wanted the whole world to know it. Second, I've used the freight elevator to follow a few. Every one of them ended up ringing the bell on thirty-two C. The occupant of that apartment is a colleague of yours, young Dr. Tunbridge Wells."

"I know him," said Keats.

"Every Saturday at four o'clock I stand in the shadows in the lobby and watch them go up in the elevator. At a quarter to six I come back and watch them walk out. It's a hobby with me, like bird watching. In England I guess they *would* call it bird watching. When the women come in they look tense and excited. When they go out, some are smiling, some are a little mussed, but they all look relaxed."

"And how did my wife look?" asked Keats with a nasty smile.

Roach turned pale. He stood up and then sat down again. "How did you find out?"

"I didn't find out. But when a super comes to me—why me?—with a cock-and-bull story about women I presumably never heard of being screwed in his apartment house, I figure it must have something to do with my family."

"It's not a cock-and-bull story, Doctor. Wells has a long line of unpaid call girls who come to his home. These women are not professionals. You should see the mink. And they're too old."

"All right, but what has this got to do with my wife?"

"She's been up twice. That's an honor. Very few of them are recalled for a repeat performance. The first time it happened, she and Wells came in together. The second time she came alone. That was when I followed her in the freight elevator. I got him to open the door by telling him that the hot water was going to be turned off. She was there, all right. I could see her handbag on the table. You don't think she was discussing the Bible, do you, the Old Testament the first time and the New Testament the second?" He coughed. "It was warm last Saturday, remember? Her coat was open. When she went up, she had on her brassiere. When she came down, she didn't. On her you can tell."

Jim raised his right fist and looked Roach in the eye. "Now I'll give you a warning. If you ever tell this to anyone, I'll break your arm. And that's only because your son is a patient of mine. If he weren't, I'd break both your arms."

"I know how you feel, believe me, Doctor. It's just that I don't like to see you played for a sucker. And don't take it too hard. My father used to say, 'A woman is only a woman, but a good cigar is a smoke.' That's from Kipling." He smiled. "My mother never liked that crack."

"Neither did Queen Victoria. That's why Kipling was never made Poet Laureate."

Roach stood up. "Don't worry, Doctor. My lips are sealed. But I'll be glad to testify for you in court whenever you want. And don't let that bastard screw you." When he reached the door, he turned around and said, "I didn't expect any thanks."

Keats called in his secretary-receptionist and told her that he did not want to see anyone or answer the telephone for fifteen minutes.

He knew that a doctor who revealed his sorrows to his patients was regarded as too emotional to practice medicine. And he agreed with the verdict. Those entrusted with comforting the sick should not add to their burdens. His thoughts returned to Wells and Annie Laurie. He remembered reading in the Bible as a little boy that the penalty for adultery was death. He had not been too sure what adultery meant, but as a doctor's son he had been pretty sure about death. Turning around in his swivel chair, he pulled out the red leather King James version he kept in the bookcase behind him. The passages he had once read were in Leviticus and Deuteronomy, he recalled. He flipped the pages in Deuteronomy. Yes, there it was, Chapter 22, Verse 22. "If a man be found lying with a woman married to an husband, then they shall both of them die, both the man that lay with the woman and the woman." Those old Israelites had the right idea, he decided. They condemned the man who argued that since he could not get it up for the old lady anymore, he was entitled to screw everything in sight, married or not, in order to preserve his virility. And they had no compassion for the woman who pleaded that she was merely seeking from another man the climax and fulfillment her husband had denied her. There were no triangles, no ménages à trois, no seventeenth-century comedies of cuckoldry, no Sun King sayings like, "A mistress a season is well within reason," and no loving thy neighbor's wife as thyself. Not on the Sinai Desert. And never any mercy, either. Just up the ass. He kept wondering how those iron-hearted Hebrews had executed a guilty pair until he saw, a little down the page, the phrase, "Ye shall stone them with stones that they die." Maybe he ought to throw a small, token rock at Wells and Annie Laurie. No? A pebble, perhaps? Oh, hell, these laws had been written thirty-three hundred years before. Still, there should be some way he could give Wells a good shot in the labonza.

What amazed him was Annie Laurie's eagerness to hop into bed. He had always thought that she disliked the sexual act even more than she disliked him. Well, he had been wrong. One thing you had to say for her, though. She was not promiscuous. Wells had been the first, he was sure, in eight years of marriage. There must be some moral statute of limitations for adultery. It was probably three years, and stated that if a wife did not go to bed with her husband during that time she was entitled to sleep with another man. Sure, sure. Only the whole thing stank. Wells was a sexual mechanic who serviced married women in return for the implied promise that they would never bother him again. Strange it was that of all men it was he who had managed to seduce Annie Laurie. The sonofabitch had stolen his wife. Soon he was going to steal his job. All that was left was the virus killer, at least three doses of it. Keats hoped that no boy whose life it would save would ever grow up to get his kicks out of screwing other men's wives. He prayed that no girl it would cure would ever develop into an intercourse-hating whore.

The secretary-receptionist knocked on the door and walked in without waiting.

"There are two patients outside. One mother is double parked. The other has a beauty-parlor appointment in forty minutes. They are stewing."

"Bring in the first one," he said.

He had never forgotten the morning he had interviewed his secretary. Before he could ask her any questions she had confessed that she did not type very well. Then she'd told him what had happened the last time she had applied for a job. The moment she had entered the huge office she had decided that she would never work there. Long rows of girls were typing as if they were puppets and the machines animated. The personnel manager was sexually aggressive and unfriendly, a combination she found disgusting. He turned her over to a nasty little woman who ushered her into a cubbyhole of an office, seated her at a desk, and told her to copy a legal document that she placed before her. The girl had used an electric typewriter only twice before. Glancing up at the woman who was standing next to her, she said, "I can't work if you keep looking over my shoulder. Do you mind waiting in that chair in the corner."

To her surprise the woman walked away and sat down. His secretary at this point began to type with blinding speed. She was not actually typing any words, merely playing on the keyboard the Clementi five-finger piano exercises she had learned so well as a child. Every time she heard a bell ring, she pressed the return bar and the carriage zipped back with an impressive noise. She was delighted to see that one of her sentences was 36k5;2'½-7=vd1Lt=Y-L= BO. As she became more confident, her speed increased. She could tell that her examiner was impressed. When the page was filled, she pulled it out, walked over to the woman in the corner, and handed her the gibberish. The moment she saw her eyes widen and her jaw sag, she said,

"All right, so nobody is perfect." As she walked out she added, "I wouldn't work for a firm that had it in for a girl just because she made a mistake in typing once in a while."

Keats had hired her on the spot.

After office hours he decided to go downtown and buy something he wanted, something extravagant. That was what Annie Laurie and other women did when they were depressed. For a long time he had been interested in small adding machines. Only they were called pocket calculators now. In the window of an electronics shop on Lexington Avenue he saw a large collection.

"I'd like to look at an inexpensive pocket calculator," he said to the salesgirl.

She lifted one from a shelf. "This is only fifty-nine fifty. It's a Kawabata."

"Where is it made?" he asked.

She turned over the device and examined it. "In Osaka."

"That's in Japan, isn't it?"

"Nah, right here in New Jersey."

"I'd like to see how it works," he said.

"What do you want to do?"

"I'd like to add three and five."

"All right," she said tolerantly, handing him the calculator. "Press the 'five' button, then the 'plus' button, then the 'three' button. Now, press this button down here."

He followed her instructions carefully. A green thirteen appeared in the little window.

"Five and three don't make thirteen," he said.

"Let me have it," she said impatiently.

She repeated what he had done. Again a green thirteen lit up the window. She shook her head. "It must be the new math."

"It's the no math," he corrected. "How do you do multiplication?"

"The same way you do addition," she replied, "only you use the 'times' sign instead of the 'plus' sign."

He took the calculator. "Let's see," he said as he began to press the buttons. "Forty-one times seventy-two." For the third time a green thirteen shone in the calculator's little window.

"Would you like to see a more expensive model?" She gave him another calculator. "This is a Doogenhouse. It's a hundred and forty-nine dollars and it's made in Detroit."

"All right," he said as he pressed some buttons. "Five plus three equals—"

A much larger and brighter green thirteen lit up the screen.

"Thank you," he said as he handed her the Doogenhouse. "These are remarkable instruments."

Just before he reached the door he turned and said, "Some afternoon I'll take you for a ride across the George Washington Bridge. To Tokyo, of course."

This was not the day to get a calculator or anything else, he decided. He made two house calls, worked an hour and a half in the Adams pediatric outpatient clinic, and then went to the medical library to read a couple of scientific periodicals. At ten minutes to five he walked into Trudy Starr's office and slumped into a chair.

"You look as if you haven't gained a yard all day," she said.

"I've just been thrown for a thirty-yard loss, and I'd like to belly-ache about it. I don't suppose you would listen to me."

"I'd love to, and right now in my apartment." She took her coat off the hanger. "I won't bother to change."

He did not realize that this was the first time she had ever left Adams in uniform.

She drove him to her apartment in her little car, which she left in the basement garage of the building. As soon as they entered the house she seated him facing the Canaletto. The view, she felt, would soothe him.

"Would you care for a drink?" she asked.

"Oh, no." He hesitated. "Maybe a Coke, if you'll have one with me."

She went to the kitchen and returned with two large glasses filled with ice and Coca-Cola. Even before she had a chance to sit down he began to tell her everything that he knew about the virus killer. Later he divulged a few things about his married life.

"Then your wife thinks you have six doses left but you only have three," she said.

He nodded. "Dr. Choate has the rest."

"Do you think he will be able to discover the formula from such a small amount?"

"No, but he has a chance of coming up with a clue. I had to give him that chance. I couldn't hog it all for myself."

"You are a generous man, Jimmy. That's why God is letting you perform these miracles."

"He's not doing much for my married life, though." He hesitated. "Annie Laurie has been unfaithful to me." He told her of the superintendent's visit, repeating almost every word he had said.

"He sounds like a slimy little voyeur," she said. "The perfect apartment-house superintendent for Wells." She shook her head. "Your colleague has a foul reputation. A couple of years ago he even tried to get the Directress of Nursing to go to bed with him. Her marriage had been shaky for some time. She claims she turned him down. If she is telling the truth, she'll regret her decision to the end of her days. He is irresistible to a certain kind of woman."

"I can't understand why his women have to be married," said Jim.

"I can't either. I once heard that his mother was an attractive and sexy woman who died in her late thirties. His father monopolized her. Neither of them paid much attention to their son. Maybe he goes around searching for a mother. When he goes to bed with one, he is so frightened at what he has done that he drops her like a hot potato."

Jim frowned. "My mother died in her thirties, too. I was nine, and I felt that she had deserted me, that if she had really loved me she would not have left me. My first wife left me, too. Her lover, who was not to be denied, was a cancer of the breast. And now, Annie Laurie. All my women leave me. I must be doing something wrong."

Trudy walked over to him, kissed him on the lips, and sat down again. "I'll never leave you."

"You're a Keats Saver," he said. "That's like a Life Saver only it tastes better."

She smiled.

"Your teeth are so white, Trudy," he said. "After a woman reaches forty, her teeth begin to turn yellow. Yours must have a thick layer of enamel."

She laughed. "You would make a remarkable lover. Instead of poetry you would quote the basic sciences. And all your compliments would be drawn from physiology and medicine."

"I'd be a faithful one." He finished the Coca-Cola. "I can't understand how Annie Laurie can be so hypocritical. After spending an afternoon in that bastard's arms, she comes home and shows a touching concern about something that she knows means a lot to me, the virus killer. She worries about its safety; she wants me to move it to my home or my office where I can keep my eye on it; she shows as much interest in its whereabouts as if she were devoted to me. It is because of her that I had a lock put on my refrigerator at Adams."

"And gave her the key. She knows where the virus killer is, and she can take it out whenever she wants. She's either very crafty or else Wells is feeding her the big idea."

"What could she do with it?" asked Jim.

"She could give it to him so that from now on he could perform the miracles. And he won't be secretive about them, like you. He will be the frank, honest, open, and aboveboard all-American young doctor who tells the trustees and the medical board exactly what he is doing with his own brand of interferon. He will probably have the nerve later on to claim that his brand is better than yours."

"I don't believe it. If that bottle is not in the refrigerator when I return from Boston, I will know that Annie Laurie is the thief. And she is smart enough to know it, too. There are only two keys and I have the other."

"Jimmy, how can you be so naive! You have to remember that Wells was trained at the Medical Center. He can pour a sterile solution from one bottle to another. He knows how to handle a syringe. Don't you see what he and your wife are going to do? As soon as you leave for the convention they will go to your lab. Your wife will open the icebox with the key you gave her and hand him the virus killer, which he will immediately pour into a bottle of his own. Then he will add saline solution to the empty bottle and replace it in the refrigerator just as it was before. After that all he has to do is lock up and walk away with your virus killer in his bag. I saw you inject it into Charlie Prince's vein. It is crystal clear and colorless, just like a saline solution. When you come back, you would never notice the difference."

"Why do you say that Annie Laurie and Wells will go to my lab together?"

"Because they don't trust each other," answered Trudy. "Would you trust either of them?"

"So you want me to put another padlock on my icebox?"

"Of course not, Jimmy. I want you to do better than that. A new padlock would only prevent Wells from stealing the virus killer. I want you to mislead them, bamboozle them, double-cross them, and catch them red-handed. Let's go to your lab right this minute. First you'll remove the virus killer from the refrigerator and put it in your little black bag. That will forever prevent them from stealing it. Your wife thinks it is in a bottle labeled 'Interferon.' So you will take any old bottle, label it 'Interferon,' sign your name under it, and squirt in twelve ml. of ordinary saline solution. Finally, you'll place this incorrectly labeled bottle in the refrigerator and lock up."

"Trudy, this is a diabolical idea. What I like best is that Wells will be stealing ordinary salt solution and replacing it with salt solution of his own."

"When you have run a department at Adams as long as I have," said Trudy, "you get to be diabolical."

"I still don't see how I can catch them red-handed, though."

"That's because you don't realize how grateful Captain Prince is. You saved Charlie's life with the virus killer. Have you forgotten that the nickname is 'Finger' Prince? The old man is head of the fingerprint division of the New York City Police Department. If I am right about all this, Wells and your wife will leave their fingerprints all over the fake interferon bottle you are going to plant in your refrigerator." She smiled. "The rest will be easy. I will get Wells's prints for you sometime this week. He drops into my office from time to time to butter me up. You can get your wife's from a clean glass at home. If Captain Prince says that the fingerprints we get for him match those on the bottle in your refrigerator, you will have done more than prove to yourself that she has sold you out to a competitor."

"I will?"

"Yes, Jimmy. You think that Wells will be the next director of Pediatrics. As things stand now, you're probably right. But if you can pin this filthy mess on him, I think you will get the job. People don't like breaking and entering, dirty tricks, and Watergating anymore."

"Suppose you're wrong? Suppose you're imagining all this?"

"Then we will have had a little fun together."

He did not say anything for a moment. "She must really love him."

"I don't think it's that at all," said Trudy.

"Then she must really hate me."

"She just doesn't give a hoot about you. I hear she is constantly telling people how much she hates to work. That doesn't do your practice any good. When she married a Park Avenue doctor, she must have thought she had it made. You've betrayed her. Besides, she doesn't want you to touch her. That shows how bad her judgment is. A woman with such poor judgment would go for any crazy scheme. She's just a patsy for Wells."

"And I suppose that what she is doing with Wells is not a betrayal of me!"

"Certainly it is, and in the modern manner. In the Victorian age a wife would give her lover her most precious possession—her virtue. But in 1973 a wife gives her lover her husband's most precious possession, in this case the virus killer. She is right about one thing, though. There is a lot of money to be made out of that miracle medicine, especially if it helps Wells get thirty-five thousand dollars a year in addition to what he makes in private practice. He must have cooked up the idea in the first place. It sounds like one of his grandiose schemes. But your wife is no fool either. I have the suspicion that when she hands him the virus killer she will be well rewarded. And not just with a roll in the hay."

She stood up. "Give me a minute to take off this uniform and put on something else." She returned in a couple of minutes in an elegant, sand-colored dress.

"You're beautiful, Trudy," he exclaimed, "and I'm not going to pull the old one by saying that this is one of the few times I've seen you with your clothes on."

"I wish it were true," she said, giving him a dazzling smile.

He stood there fascinated.

"I think you like me for my thick layer of enamel," she added with a sigh.

They took a taxi to Adams. As was usually the case at this hour, the research laboratories were empty. The door to Jim's room was guarded by the dog, who nuzzled Trudy's thighs as soon as she walked up to him.

Jim smiled. "This is a highly intelligent animal. He knows a good pair of thighs when he sees one."

He unlocked the refrigerator, took out a bottle labeled "Interferon," and handed it to her. "Keep this for me."

"I've never been entrusted with anything so valuable in my life. Not even the pictures."

"I have to trust you because of your name," he said. "The first three letters of Trudy and the first two letters of Starr spell 'trust.'"

While she was carefully putting the virus killer in her handbag he sat down at a beat-up portable on a desk in the corner, typed the word *interferon* in capital letters on a gummed label, and signed his name. Then he affixed the label to an empty, sterile bottle he brought down from a shelf just above his head. Finally he reached into a drawer for a large, disposable syringe with a needle attached and a bottle of sterile saline solution, both of which he placed on the metal table.

"Give me a hand, Trudy," he said as he plunged the needle through the rubber diaphragm of the bottle containing the saline solution.

He inverted the bottle and handed it to her.

"You're going to take out twelve ml., aren't you?" she asked. "That's what they expect to find."

He nodded, drew out the exact amount, and pulled out the syringe. "Throw the saline into the trash basket," he said. "Now unscrew the cap on the empty bottle and hold it in front of me."

As soon as he transferred the saline she screwed on the cap, carefully wiped the entire bottle with a clean towel, and placed it in the refrigerator. "That should put an end to their criminal career."

"Maybe they will never enter this lab," he said as he attached the padlock to the "eye" bolts. "If they do, I would like to be here and invisible when Wells takes out our saline solution and replaces it with his own."

"God will be here and invisible. And He has a great sense of humor. Whoever created Tunbridge Wells must have a great sense of humor, and always the last laugh."

As they walked out together the dog nuzzled her thighs again.

"I see I have a rival," said Jim.

"Yes, you do," she answered, glancing up at his head, "and so far he has the inside track. But that's only because he's bolder than you and has more hair."

They rode down in an empty elevator.

"Don't feel too bad," she said. "You haven't lost anything. You never had her."

"How do you rate old and penniless pediatricians?"

"Number one," she answered.

As he helped her into the taxi she turned and said, "If you get lonesome in Boston, call me."

"I'm lonesome already," he said.

The next morning Wells decided that if he was going to give Annie a check for thirty-five thousand dollars the following night, he had better verify her story. He telephoned Tugend in the research laboratories.

"I wonder whether you would do me a favor."

"Certainly, Herr Doktor," said the animal keeper, who knew that Wells, a great favorite of the Director of Laboratories, would undoubtedly be the next director of Pediatrics.

"Then meet me in the animal room in half an hour."

Knowing Tugend's fondness for good cigars. Wells bought a box of Corona Coronas on the way to Adams. As soon as he walked into the little office just off the animal room, he said,

"A patient of mine just brought me some Corona Coronas. I don't smoke, and I was hoping that a connoisseur would smoke them for me." He handed Tugend the gift-wrapped box.

"Is that the favor?" exclaimed the animal keeper.

"That's it," said Wells.

"Thank you, Herr Doktor. You are *ein gebildeter Mann,* a true gentleman."

Recently the use of German was becoming more fashionable, he was glad to see. He took especial pleasure in using his old language again now that even Willy Brandt, the socialist, was turning against Israel. They ought to cover that accursed country with six feet of Saudi Arabian oil and set fire to it.

"I can see why Dr. Grant thinks so highly of you," he added.

"I understand that you are practicing advanced veterinary medicine up here," said Wells with a smile. "I hear that someone cured one of your animals, a dog, I believe, of a bad case of distemper."

"Not a bad case, a fatal case. I am a good animal man and I tell you that nothing in the world could have saved that dog. But Dr. Keats did. How can you account for that? Only one way. He used a secret remedy of his, something nobody has ever heard of. He just put a padlock on the icebox in his laboratory. Why would a doctor do a thing like that? And I caught him once with his sleeve rolled up and a syringe on the table next to him. I don't know what he injected into himself, but right after that some warts he had had for a long time disappeared one-two-three, by magic. And a terrible cold, too. It's all a big mystery. But he is a strange man, a violent and dangerous man, so there is nothing you can do to find out."

Wells waved and walked away. As soon as he reached his office he rang Annie Laurie at work to get the name of the little girl with chickenpox pneumonia whose life Keats had saved. There were fifty-eight Rushes in the Manhattan telephone book, but only one lived on Park Avenue. To Mrs. Rush, who answered the telephone herself, he explained that he was from the *New York Times* and was in the process of compiling a big article on progress in medicine for the Sunday edition. He was calling for information about the remarkable cure of her daughter's recent illness. As soon as he assured her that no names would be mentioned, she told him everything about the case, including her opinion of doctors who played around with supernatural remedies. Just before he thanked her and hung up, he asked her if the pediatrician was Dr. James Keats. She assured him that he was indeed.

That afternoon, after seeing twenty-two patients in his office, he drove up to the Medical Center in his baby blue 1974 Cadillac Eldorado. When discussing cases with the fourteen pediatric residents at Adams, he often referred to the Medical Center as his old stamping-grounds. This time he went directly to the virology laboratory looking for a slim-hipped technician he had slept with when he was a pediatric resident and she newly married. She seemed delighted and flattered by his visit. The small sterile bottle he asked for she handed him at once.

He looked around the room. "Things must have changed since I was chief resident," he said. "I hear one of your male technicians went berserk recently."

"Not from overwork. All he had to do was pour out a little interferon for some doctor from Adams. Right after that he started to wreck the joint. The police had to take him away. Dr. Choate was very nice about it, though."

She took his hand. "I have had two children since we were together that night. I'm much bigger inside now. Why don't you try me again. You might find the comparison interesting. My husband does."

He smiled and took his hand away. "Ring me when you've given birth to two more."

On the way back to his office he reflected that Ann's story had been accurate. She would make a good ally. And at thirty-five thousand dollars the virus killer might prove to be a bargain. True it was that he himself performed miracles in his office every day for pin money, but nobody paid any attention to them. For twenty dollars or less he, like every other pediatrician, prevented a child from getting whooping cough, diphtheria, lockjaw, and polio, and threw in a free physical examination as well. When it came to fees, though, pediatricians were the low men on the totem pole, the prat boys of medicine. Other specialties were less idealistic. Urologists were getting two thousand dollars for a prostatectomy, an operation that was as old as the hills, required no unusual skills, and had been performed successfully hundreds of thousands of times. With this fee in mind, he asked himself how much a tycoon father of a dying child would be willing to pay for an injection of the virus killer after he had been told by a battery of eminent consultants that the patient was doomed without it. And especially if he learned that there were fewer than half a dozen doses left in the world. Wells smiled as he thought of a figure.

At precisely nine o'clock the following night he walked through the lobby of the hospital wearing his white coat and carrying his little black bag. Annie Laurie was just coming through the main entrance. They nodded to each other and moved separately toward the elevator. When they reached the seventh floor she got out just ahead of him. As he had guessed, no one was in the research laboratories. They had no difficulty finding Keats's darkened room. Perhaps because he was so anxious to get to the refrigerator, Wells stepped on the sleeping dog's tail. The animal yelped, jumped up in alarm, and tore a large piece out of his tormentor's trouser cuff. Annie Laurie turned on the light.

"Get out of here, you nasty beast," she cried, trying to keep her voice down.

The dog gave her an aggrieved look and trotted out to the corridor. She closed the door.

"It's my favorite suit," said Wells. It was certainly his flashiest, a distinctive, light-plaid, made-to-order model.

"Don't fret," said Annie Laurie, delighted to be able to use a phrase he had used on her. "There's a place around the corner from you that does expert weaving. When they get finished, the suit will be as good as new."

He looked around him quickly. "Let's get the refrigerator open," he said.

She smiled. "That's why I'm here. But first let me have the check."

He reached into his breast pocket, brought out a check, and handed it to her. She examined it carefully, as if she expected to be tricked. It was certified, and made out to her for thirty-five thousand dollars. She folded it, put it into her handbag, and came out with the key.

"Do you have to be such a lady, Ann," he said. "Take off your gloves. You might have to help me, you know."

She pulled off her gloves and stuffed them in her purse. As she expected, she had no difficulty in unfastening the padlock. When she swung open the refrigerator door, she saw at once a small bottle labeled "Interferon" on the top shelf. Underneath the typewritten word, as if to verify its authenticity, was her husband's signature. She grasped the bottle firmly to prevent her hand from shaking and gave it to Wells.

"Just a minute," he said. "Let me look through that refrigerator myself."

It contained only three petri dishes and a flask of Hank's solution. He glanced at the bottle he was holding.

"It's the real McCoy," he said as he closed the door. "Now let me show you how we do things at the Medical Center." He seemed more relaxed.

He put Keats's labeled bottle on the metal table, took the empty one he had obtained from the Medical Center technician out of his black bag, and placed them side by side. After unscrewing both caps, he lit the Bunsen burner, flamed the mouths of the two bottles to preserve sterility, and with a steady hand poured what he imagined was the virus killer from Keats's labeled bottle into his own. The latter he capped at once. Again he reached into his black bag, this time coming out with a disposable syringe and a one-hundred-ml. bottle of sterile saline solution. With a little help from Annie Laurie, he removed exactly twelve ml. of the solution and squirted it into the now empty bottle that he had just taken out of the refrigerator. After screwing on the cap, he stepped back and compared the two bottles.

"They look exactly alike," he said with a smile.

It would have been surprising if they had not since they both contained ordinary salt solution.

The unlabeled bottle he wedged into his bag in an upright position. The one with Keats's signature he replaced in the refrigerator. He closed the door gently and snapped on the padlock. Looking around the room to be sure that they had left nothing there, he motioned her to go ahead of him, and said,

"Jesse James in his heyday couldn't have done a better job. We're off in a cloud of heifer dust."

"I just hope that beast is not lurking in the corridor waiting to tear off a piece of your other trouser cuff. He might go in for matched pairs, like Frick with his pictures in that wonderful museum on Seventieth Street."

"Come on, Ann! We'll worry about the dog and the Frick Museum and the state of the union when we get downstairs."

As soon as they reached the street he said, "Can you come up to my apartment?"

"I don't think I'd better."

"I know, you have to go home and cook. Oh well, why don't you come with me and simmer, smolder, and flame. It will be much more fun for both of us."

"All right, but I have to be home at midnight in case Jim rings up from Boston."

"That's okay, Cinderella. If the prince in the fairy tale could put up with such behavior, so can I. I'll even drive you home in a car that General Motors guarantees will not turn into a pumpkin at midnight."

After a moment he asked, "Are you taking the pill?"

Her face tightened. "I don't have to."

Jim did not ring her up that night or any other night. He did, however, telephone Trudy regularly. They arranged to meet in his laboratory at nine o'clock Saturday morning. When she walked in five minutes early carrying a large manila envelope, she found him staring at a piece of plaid cloth he held in his hand.

She smiled at him and asked, "Were they here?"

He held up the material. "Do you recognize this? I found it between the dog's paws when I came in this morning."

"Of course. It's from Tunbridge Wells's flashy suit."

"Right. It's too bad the animal didn't take his foot off."

"What about the refrigerator?"

"I haven't opened it yet."

"Open it. I can't wait." She gave a mock sigh of satisfaction. "This is our first date."

He unfastened the padlock with his key and swung open the refrigerator door. "I think the bottle has been moved. You left it perfectly straight. Now it's at a fifteen-degree angle."

Using a towel to lift it by the neck, he placed it on the metal table. "I don't see any prints," he said.

"I didn't see any on my dolphin, either."

"Let's try the experimental method," he said.

He took an empty bottle from the shelf, wiped it carefully with a towel, and pressed his fingertips against it. "No prints," he said. "I guess they have to be brought out by experts."

He sat down at the little table in the corner and typed on a tag, "This bottle was found in the refrigerator of the research laboratory of Dr. James Keats on 10 November, 1973 at 9 A.M."

After Trudy and he had signed their names beneath the inscription, he tied the tag around the neck of the bottle and slid it into a manila envelope.

"I'll feel like an ass," he said, "if after we've laid this elaborate trap we find that they were frightened away by the dog."

"Not your wife," said Trudy.

She opened the manila envelope she had brought. "This is my contribution to the cause."

"What cause?"

"Keats for director. I'm Chairwoman of the Women's Campaign Committee."

"And how many members do you have?"

"One, me."

With her handkerchief she removed a sleek, glass, four-inch dolphin and placed it on the metal table.

"It's beautiful, Trudy."

"Yes, it's Steuben glass. Two or three times a week Wells comes to my office to pay court to me. He knows that I am impervious to his matinee-idol charms, but he nevertheless feels he must placate me since he regards me more as a kind of powerful tribal goddess than an Adams landmark. When he saw the statuette on my desk, he praised it extravagantly. I remarked that it was much heavier than it seemed. He responded at once by lifting it, weighing it in his hand, and fondling it. And, of course, by agreeing with me."

She tied a signed tag to the statuette and returned it to the envelope. "A dolphin for the captain. How about your wife's prints?"

"I have them on a glass."

After morning hours he telephoned Captain Prince, who promised to come to the office at five that afternoon. When he arrived with Count of Monte Cristo promptness, he found the doctor tired and drawn. As soon as they were seated, Jim said,

"The drug I injected into Charlie's vein was a virus killer of unknown composition. Until its formula is discovered, it can never be duplicated. That might take twenty years or half a century. And there are only three doses left."

"I am more grateful than ever. I hope you've kept it under lock and key."

"Yes, I did, in a bottle labeled 'Interferon' in my refrigerator at Adams." He hesitated. "I think that someone poured out the contents of that bottle for himself and put salt solution in the original container."

"That's a felony, Doctor. Who do you think did it?"

"A young Adams pediatrician called Tunbridge Wells."

"A rival?"

"Yes, in more ways than one. We are both coming up for the same job, chief of Pediatrics."

"Do you mean to tell me he sawed through the lock? Or picked it?"

Keats shook his head.

"Well then who has a key to the refrigerator besides you?" asked the captain.

"Only my wife."

"I see." The captain looked grave. "You want me to get the virus killer back, is that it? You realize that it will be very unpleasant for your wife and Dr. Wells if I do."

Keats gave a mirthless laugh. "No, no! I don't want you to do anything of the kind. I took the bottle with the virus killer out of the icebox myself some time ago and substituted another one with saline solution in it. If things worked out the way I think they did, all Wells got was some ordinary salt solution."

The captain gave Jim a hard look. "Doctor, you're a foxy grandpa, a regular fancy Dan. You never used to be like that when you played football, just boom through right tackle for five yards. Do you think your wife and Wells have been intimate?"

"I know they have been."

The captain shrugged. "Then maybe your natural jealousy has made you imagine too much. What would you like me to do?"

Jim took three manila envelopes out of his desk drawer. "The bottle in here labeled 'Interferon' was carefully wiped off, signed by me, and put in my refrigerator just before I went to Boston for three days. The glass in here has my wife's prints all over it; the dolphin in here, Dr. Wells's. I would like to find out if the fingerprints on the bottle that was in my locked refrigerator belong to my wife and Dr. Wells."

"You shall, Doctor, and soon. But maybe there won't be any fingerprints on the bottle. That would be better for all concerned, believe me."

At eleven o'clock Monday morning Captain Prince telephoned Jim. "There are two sets of prints on the bottle. One matches those on a drinking glass labeled 'Annie Laurie Keats.' The other is identical with those on a glass statue of a dolphin labeled 'Tunbridge Wells.' I am sending you an unofficial report, and I will testify in court when the time comes. It's still a felony, Doctor. I'm sorry about the whole thing, but sometimes it all turns out for the best."

"It may at that. Thanks. And tell Charlie that someday I'll make a fullback out of him, or a doctor, or both. You don't know how lucky you are to have a good wife and a good son."

"I wouldn't have a son if it weren't for you."

12

BY ONE THIRTY that afternoon, "Caries" Grant and Evan Dummer had been waiting for their two colleagues for almost half an hour, sipping beer and talking about Adams at a corner table in Jaegers Restaurant, where they could not be overheard.

"I wonder what's holding them up," said Dummer.

"Their big practices," replied Grant.

Five minutes later Akt and Bligh walked in, murmured their regrets, and sat down. Everyone had Dortmunder dunkeles and sauerbraten. Just before coffee, Akt tapped on the table with his spoon and said,

"Gentlemen, as president of the medical board, I call this meeting of the majority to order."

"To the democratic process," said Bligh, raising his stein with his left hand. Even so, a little beer spilled over.

The waiter placed coffee before them. Dummer asked for Sanka.

"I don't deny," said Courtney Akt, "that Keats is a competent pediatrician, but people just can't work with him. He is too abrasive. There is no give and take. He would be the impossible chief. To show you what I mean, in the early fifties I sent him a little work. I felt sorry for him. He didn't have much of a practice and he had been to war. I hadn't. After all, what use would an obstetrician and gynecologist have been?" he asked rhetorically, raising his hands palms upward and conveniently forgetting that there were WACS, WAVES, and nurses in the armed forces. "Naturally, I didn't send him any rich or famous patients. They would never have taken their babies to an unknown pediatrician anyway. But I did recommend him to some good little people in Washington Heights, Brooklyn, and the Bronx. At the end of a year and a half, what do you think he did? One day he got hold of me in the doctors' lounge, made me sit down, and handed me a sheet of paper on which had been typed the names and addresses of nineteen patients I had referred to him who had not paid their bills. You won't believe this, but he asked me not to send him any more normal newborns if the fathers were deadbeats. Good patients, he informed me, he would be glad to accept any time." The mandarin moon-face, until then so serene, now clouded. "That was twenty years ago, and I've never sent him another patient since. Was it my fault that they didn't pay him? How can you work with a man like that?"

"If he gets the job," said Bligh, "he will make a shambles out of the hospital in three months. Take pediatric cardiology, for instance. It is doing quite nicely under Holden, the Department of Pediatrics cooperative cardiologist. Of course, I realize that in effect it has become a part of Surgery. But Dummer, a wise bird if there ever was one, knows this and has given us his blessing. You see, in the old days, most heart disease in children was rheumatic in origin. Now, most is congenital. And the treatment for that, if there is any treatment in a particular case, is operation. As the art and science of surgery progresses, more and more such patients will come under the knife. In Adams today, pediatric cardiology really belongs to Surgery. Oh, I know, officially and in the yearly report it is listed under the Department of Pediatrics. And so it should be. But when the chips are down, it's got to be managed and controlled by us. As Frank Ray would say, de jure it's under Pediatrics; de facto under Surgery. Evan has been most helpful."

"I try to be accommodating," said Dummer.

"But Keats, the former famous football star," continued the Director of Surgery, "has different ideas. He has spread the word around that if he is ever made director of Pediatrics, the first thing he will do is throw out Holden and appoint a pediatric cardiologist who will be loyal to the Department of Pediatrics. He tells people that in every university hospital in the country pediatric cardiology comes under its department of pediatrics. We all know that. But Adams is not every university hospital in the country. We have our own system. I'll tell you this. If that man were ever elected to the medical board, this hospital would never have another peaceful moment again. He's a congenital troublemaker."

"And insulting besides," said Grant. "Power would go to his head. What gets me, though, is the way he sits in that crummy little lab of his every day turning out so-called research that nobody pays any attention to. He would never discuss it with me, the Director of Laboratories. Oh no, why should he? He knows it all. The fact that I could give him a tip here and there cuts no ice with him."

"In all fairness," said Dummer, "I have to admit that he discusses his work with me. I let him go ahead because it keeps him out of mischief."

"Sure, and in all fairness I have to admit that he turns out a lot of papers," said Grant. "Do you know why? Because his practice is so small he has nothing else to do. You don't see Bridge Wells writing articles. He's too busy taking care of his patients."

"Many of whom he refers to appropriate specialists here at Adams," said Bligh. "He has sent me some fascinating cases in the past three years."

"If Keats got the job," said Dummer, "my group of fourteen residents would wither away. He antagonizes them. He says they don't do any work. He's always talking about Bridge Wells and his fourteen drones. I'm afraid Keats's big trouble is that he can't get along with the people who count."

Bligh tried to spear an olive from the bowl the waiter had left on the table, but his tremor was so great that he transferred the fork from his right hand to his left.

"That's only one of his faults," he said with a sweet and sour smile. "He is infatuated with the past, with ancestor worship, and the father image. His idea of medical education is drudgery for the young. We have to elect somebody with a forward-looking philosophy. We can't have a man running the Department of Pediatrics who is constantly looking over his shoulder in the hope that the old days will still be there."

"Let's stop this preaching to the converted," said Courtney Akt irritably, tapping on the table with his spoon and looking at his wristwatch as if he were going to pick up his brother at Kennedy Airport at any moment. "The four of us are going to vote for Wells. That's settled. We all know it. The question is whether our votes will be enough. If Airov goes along with the everlasting minority, Ray and Scotti, the vote will be four to three. The trustees will never let such a squeaker pass, not for a directorship. If Airov sides with us, the vote will be five to two. That might slide by."

"Maybe," said Grant.

"What you seem to have forgotten," Akt continued, "is that for years now we have been running the hospital, and on five-to-two and four-to-three ballots. And we haven't done so bad a job at that. Let us for a moment imagine the unimaginable. Suppose that on Dummer's retirement Keats were to be chosen chief. He would never vote with us. The lineup would then be Keats, Scotti, and Ray on one side; we three, Bligh, Grant, and myself, on the other. That leaves Airov. He could easily vote with them."

Dummer asked the waiter for more Sanka. He was being ignored.

"What is at stake here," Akt went on, "is control of the hospital. We could easily lose it."

"Somebody has to lean on Airov," said Grant. "An anesthetist makes his living from surgeons. Bligh, you're elected."

"Very well," said Bligh, "I'll twist his arm."

Scotti and Ray were having lunch at O'Dowd's, whose high ceilings and innumerable windows gave the radiologist the illusion that he was breathing easily once more. After having served him for twenty years, John O'Dowd knew better than anyone how much the cancer of the lung and the cobalt therapy had diminished his customer's appetite. He also realized how damaging to morale it was for a once-hungry doctor to leave three quarters of the food on his plate untouched. The proprietor therefore insisted on recommending to him the secret specials of the day. These actually consisted of a very small portion of anything that was on the menu. By the end of the meal the radiologist's plate was usually empty. And he was delighted to see how inexpensive the specials always were.

"Before I die next year," said Ray, "maybe we can win a couple of battles on the medical board. You must have read about the stuffed shirts in the United States Supreme Court who used to hand down those reactionary decisions in the twenties and thirties. They always seemed to end, 'Holmes and Brandeis dissenting.' Some people are saying that we have become the Holmes and Brandeis of the medical board. It's very flattering but it's also damned frustrating."

"We have the integrity. They have the votes," said Scotti. "Would you like to switch?"

"No, but I would like to have both," said Ray. He coughed into his handkerchief. "You know, John, patients with carcinoma of the lung have lasted two or three years. Maybe I will."

"I'm counting on it," said Scotti.

"If we could win control, there are a few things I would like to do. I'd like to cut the house staff in half, thus saving the hospital almost a million dollars a year, and ensuring that the remaining residents would do a full day's work. I would like to be able to say to them, 'Forget your television image. Remember that your four years at Adams are an extension of medical school, that you are receiving expert instruction, practical teaching, experience, and living quarters all free of charge. We demand no tuition fee from you. Quite the contrary, we pay some of you eighteen thousand dollars a year. For this salary we now demand that you do at least five thousand dollars' worth of work a year.' Believe me, John, if we could get them to give us that much, it would be a great improvement."

He tried unsuccessfully to control his cough. "I would like to do something about the inadequate nursing and floor care the patients are getting for the one hundred and seventy dollars a day in private and their one hundred dollars a day on the so-called free wards. I would like to be able to say to some of our employees, 'Give us for the one hundred and sixty dollars a week we are now paying you what you once gave us for fifteen.' I would like to be able to do something about the administrators and the inefficient efficiency experts who see dollar signs where we see patients. I would like to do something about the sneaky waste, and the thousands of unnecessary tests that are performed to appease and educate the residents. I would like to see a research division created which would transform Adams from a humdrum purveyor of routine care to an institution in which the present is married to the future. I would like to see so many beds added that a deserving case is never turned away again, so that no one with heart failure, a bleeding gastric ulcer, a cancer, or a stroke is ever put on a five-day waiting list while the money-obsessed administrators of our city recite in unison the greatest non-sequitur of modern times, 'The bed capacity of the hospitals in New York must be reduced.' I would like to help change a system in which a man walks out of Adams after sixty days owing the doctor who saved his life nine hundred dollars and the hospital which made him wait half an hour for a bedpan twelve thousand. The people won't stand for this much longer."

"You'll be around, Frank. I see you've cleaned up your plate."

"If we could get Jim Keats elected maybe I could make a start. On the basis of ability he would win hands down. But ability is no longer what counts at Adams. Wells is nothing but a young super-salesman with a big prick who has bamboozled the mothers and impressed a lot of people at Adams who know even less about medicine than he does. He has never published anything in his life. He deserves to be made director of Pediatrics as much as a high-school drum majorette deserves to be made dean of Vassar."

Scotti nodded. "I've known Jim Keats since college. We played football together. That's when you learn a lot about a man. He's worked his ass off for Adams for thirty years, and he would still be doing it if Dummer and Wells had let him. He has written more scientific papers than the entire Department of Pediatrics put together. Before Wells and Dummer effectively banished their attending staff from the service because they couldn't stand the competition, his four-times-a-week rounds were as brilliant, as exciting, yes, and as theatrical as Rintman's at McKinley or Libman's at Mt. Sinai. He is an outstanding doctor. Nobody in any specialty, and I include myself, has his clinical eye. And he's a scholar and a master of the medical literature. Any hospital would be lucky to have him. Adams doesn't deserve him."

"If we could get him elected," said Ray, beginning to look a little wistful, "and I admit it would take divine intervention, he would certainly vote with us. Since he would take Dummer's place, that would make it three against three, we against Grant, Bligh, and President Akt. Everything would then depend on Airov." He smiled. "It would be fun to be on the winning side for a little while."

"Don't forget that Dummer still has a vote," said Scotti. "Even if we could persuade Airov to vote with us, it would still be four to three in favor of Wells."

"Yes, but that's too close to slip by the board of trustees. Maybe something would happen. We would at least have a chance."

"Maybe we ought to talk to Airov," said Scotti.

"I think it would be a mistake," said Ray. "Underneath the charm, the grace, the handsome virility, and the unwillingness to relinquish an entrancing Russian accent, there is a very tough muzhik. We would only get his back up. Let the other side try."

During the early part of the week several members of the Department of Surgery intercepted Airov in the corridors and, rather clumsily, he thought, lectured him on Wells's importance to the hospital. This advance party was soon replaced by a number of more aggressive senior surgeons who one by one and without laying any foundation asked him point blank how he was going to vote. Airov was incensed. Such a question addressed to a member of the medical board by a nonmember had always been tabu. In the past, the busy-body would have been branded a dolt and made to pay for his effrontery. But Airov did not reveal his anger. When questioned he would flash his big peasant smile, shrug his shoulders, and say, "There is an old Russian proverb which goes . . ." Here he would mumble a few words in his mother tongue and walk away, a simple, hulking fellow. At last a pugnacious member of Bligh's staff caught him as he was coming out of the operating room and said,

"A lot of us on the surgical service would like to know whether you are going to vote for Wells. This time just answer yes or no."

Airov gave him his broad, guileless smile, shrugged, and said, "In my country there is an old saying which goes . . ." Then he mumbled a few words in Russian.

"In English what does the mumbo-jumbo mean?" asked the surgeon.

Suddenly the simple serf with the obsequious smile was replaced by a hard-faced and very tough muzhik.

"It means," said Airov in remarkably accent-free English, "up yours!"

After that no one on the surgical service ever mentioned Wells to him again. No one, that is, except the director. The following week Bligh asked to see him in the little office off the main operating room.

"Leonid, we think it important that Wells be made the new director of Pediatrics. We don't want to retreat into the past with Keats. He's a good pediatrician, but he would never fit into our club. And the medical board is a club. We have the usual majority, but this time it won't be enough. With your vote we think it would be. We're counting on it."

Airov turned his handsome head away from Bligh for a moment. "I was fifty-one when I was made director. Wells is thirty-eight. Can't he wait?" He seemed to be reminiscing. "There is an old Russian proverb which goes, 'A miracle is a man-made marvel which is dedicated to God.'" This saying had never been heard in the Soviet Union because Airov had just thought it up. "Suppose a man-made miracle did take place and Keats was elected director. The medical board would be split down the middle with you, Grant, and Akt on one side; Scotti, Ray, and Keats on the other. I would be the swing man. You have had your gallon of power. Why shouldn't I have my dram?"

"So you are determined to vote for Keats?"

"Right now I'm not determined to vote for anyone. The day of the meeting I'll see."

Bligh broke out into his sweet-and-sour smile. "Anesthesiology is a parasite's specialty, Leonid. You live off the surgeon. All your patients are referred to you by surgeons. I should hate to have to stop sending you work and to suggest to my loyal staff that they follow my example."

Tears came to Airov's eyes, but they were tears of laughter. When he stopped shaking he said, "I am a rich man. My family has always been very rich. And my wife is even wealthier. We don't have to worry where our next tin of caviar is coming from. You mustn't think us hard up just because we eat sevruga every night and save the beluga molossol for the big occasions. I have nine more years at Adams, and I intend to stay here until exactly midnight on my sixty-fifth birthday. My wife, a truly formidable woman, will see to it that I do. She should not find it too difficult since she knows so many of the trustees' wives intimately. And even if I never do another case for you and your sycophants, I will enjoy myself during those nine years by talking against and voting against every measure you bring up."

"Leonid, Leonid!"

"Just a moment, please. When your boys get the really tough ones, the life-or-death cases, which anesthetist will they turn to? When you have one of your seven-hour block dissections, whom will you ask to put the mask on the patient? Me? Maybe I will be busy. Maybe I will say that you're a turtle, that my job is to put people to sleep, not to fall asleep myself at the table. Maybe I'll say that I know of cases in which a localized cancer metastasized through the patient's body by the time you finished because you dragged your feet."

"Leonid, I'm just trying to do what's best for the hospital."

Airov responded with his big laugh. "You're just trying to do what's best for Bligh."

13

TOM GUTHRIE had always been smart. The son of a brilliant but unsuccessful West Side general practitioner and a devout Scotch Presbyterian mother, each equally responsible for his high I.Q., he had won a scholarship to an exclusive Manhattan private school and then another to the Wharton School of Business. His rise had been rapid. At fifty he was a millionaire many times over and chairman of the board of Guthrie and Co., respected Wall Street investment bankers. His mother had continually preached to him that after every financial success he should contribute something to a good cause. On the other hand, she was equally firm in telling him that the period after an unfortunate business venture was not the time to give to charity. She was obviously trying to effect a Pavlovian conditioning of God. Whenever He looked down and saw that one of His charities needed money, she reasoned, He would automatically be nice to her boy. Fortunately for Adams, her son had heeded her advice. And during the six years he had been on the board of trustees, he had never suffered a financial reverse.

When he was thirty-three he married Lydia, seven years younger than he, an impoverished member of a very old New York family. Although she did not become pregnant during the first years of their marriage, her apparent sterility did not interfere with its success. She had beauty, grace, and now that she had money, friends. Her barrenness she and her husband had used as an excuse for an amazingly active sex life. Their secret motto became, "If at first you don't conceive, try, try again!" At last the perseverance which they had both found so enjoyable was rewarded. On their sixth wedding anniversary an eight-and-a-half-pound son was born. He was christened DeWitt after an eighteenth-century landholding ancestor of Lydia's. But everyone called him Corky because his paternal grandfather, the old doctor, would gaze at him in admiration and say, "He's a corker!"

The baby thrived. When he was a year old he weighed twenty-six pounds and walked quite well. At that time his pediatrician, a doctor from the Medical Center who had taken care of Lydia as a child, told her to be sure to bring him back the following month for his inoculation against measles. She failed to keep her appointment. A few months later while making a house call because Corky had a febrile upper-respiratory infection, he again warned her to get the boy protected. Shortly after this he could warn her no more. He had dropped dead with a cardiac infarction. The pediatrician who took over his practice had difficulty deciphering his colleague's almost illegible handwriting. Seated across the desk from Lydia, who had just brought her son to the office because of a mild stomach upset, he asked as he put down the chart,

"Has the little fellow been protected against measles?"

Lydia, remembering the many shots he had received, smiled and said, "He's been protected against everything."

In truth her mind was elsewhere. Her husband had just bought her a beautiful place in Vermont. An expert rider, she had soon joined the local hunt club whose members were not only socially prominent but humane as well. Most of them did not believe in killing animals except for food. There were even a few vegetarians on the roster. They resolved the conflict between their compassion and the rigorous rules of the hunt by keeping two foxes in an enclosure far from the clubhouse. It was soon discovered that the depositing of wads of cotton waste within the pen would induce the animals to void upon them. The morning of the hunt, the keeper would collect these urine-impregnated lumps and stuff them into a net bag which he would attach to the rear of a Land Rover. Assembled in front of the clubhouse would be the hounds and the hunters on their sleek horses. The master of the hunt would always give the automobile a sporting head start. Then, at a blast of his horn, the pack would leap forward and unerringly follow the scent of the fox urine. The driver of the Land Rover and his observer for their part would not take advantage of the pack. They traveled at about the same speed as the average fast fox. The huntsmen and huntswomen rode beautifully, crossing fields, clearing hedges, and occasionally trampling on a flowerbed or a cabbage patch just as they would have if they had been pursuing an animal. In addition to its humanity, this system allowed the members to determine exactly how long the hunt would last. If the master said that today it would last three quarters of an hour, the driver and his observer, by speeding up and slowing down their automobile, would see to it that the hounds, baying furiously, would surround the Land Rover in exactly forty-five minutes. Then came the climax of the day. A member specially chosen for the honor would cut the urine-impregnated bag from the automobile and toss it to the pack, who would smell it suspiciously and not know what to do with it. In this way the club enjoyed the pleasures of the hunt without having to witness its grisly ending. Lydia never missed a weekend performance. And Corky never received his measles inoculation.

He grew up to be a golden boy, handsome, brave, and kind. He consistently surpassed the distinguished record his father had once compiled in the very school he now attended. When he was eleven, the headmaster told Tom Guthrie that his son had an I.Q. of a hundred seventy and was the finest student who had ever passed through his hands. He was a good athlete as well, particularly in track and basketball. But his passion was riflery. He attained scores on the range that crack shots of sixteen envied.

His paternal grandmother doted on him. She visited him frequently even though she did not approve of what she regarded as the loose moral tone of the household. Without having any proof, she felt that the sexual life of her son and daughter-in-law was far too active to her way of thinking. On her own marriage night she had informed her husband that she would have relations with him twice a week, no more and no less, and that she expected him to keep to this schedule until death parted them. He was seventy-seven now and he still had sexual intercourse with her twice a week. That was what made him a good man, she felt, stamina and consistency. Lydia's fox hunting she branded immoral because it was false. Voyeurism she held in contempt because it was so wasteful. A good erection should be put to use. Shortly after the Metropolitan Museum of Art bought Rembrandt's *Aristotle Contemplating the Bust of Homer* for four and a half million dollars, a friend of Tom's who was both a wag and a member of the firm brought two statues to the Guthries' home. One, about twelve inches high, was a replica of the Venus de Milo. The other, about eight inches in height, was a statue of Aristotle. The banker placed them facing each other so that the philosopher's eyes were on a level with the enticing torso of the Queen of Love. On the table he placed a card which read, "Aristotle Contemplating the Bust of Venus." Every time Grandma Guthrie visited Corky, the first thing she did was to walk briskly to the table and turn the statue of Aristotle around so that he would no longer be able to gaze so outrageously at the goddess's naked charms. She was persistent. On every occasion she tried to impress on her grandson, as she had on her son, her own stern code of morality. But Corky loved her because he felt that underneath the preaching there was a warm and earthy woman.

After Tom Guthrie had been an Adams trustee for a few years Lydia suggested to him that they change pediatricians. She felt that it was disloyal of them to have someone from another hospital.

"Everyone is going to Tunbridge Wells," she said.

Her husband looked dubious. "If you want to go to him to show our loyalty to Adams, fine. But if you're making the change because he's a handsome philanderer, the answer is no."

Lydia smiled. "One handsome philanderer in the family is enough."

"I'm not a philanderer," said her husband indignantly, denying on the one hand her accusation of infidelity while accepting on the other her assessment of his looks.

"I know. But you would be if I didn't keep you so busy."

He seemed disinclined to pursue the conversation, but at last he said, "My mother has met Wells several times. She doesn't like him at all."

In spite of her mother-in-law's opinion, Lydia changed pediatricians. And she took Corky for routine check-ups and booster injections far more frequently than ever before. When he was eleven he suddenly came down with a high fever and an intractable cough. If Wells had looked at the inside of his patient's cheeks while he was examining the throat, he would have seen Koplik spots, those telltale forerunners of oncoming measles. His oversight made little difference, however. Three days later the rash which suddenly appeared was so typical that the diagnosis was no longer in doubt. He was too shrewd to ask why the boy had never been inoculated against the disease. Lydia's ill-concealed sense of guilt warned him away from this line of questioning. Besides, he was delighted that she did not reproach him for overlooking the injection. Instead, he reassured her that the case was of average severity with no complications. Corky made a rapid recovery and went back to school in two weeks.

That term was his most successful. He far outdistanced the pupils in his form. In addition, he made the junior varsity basketball team. But his greatest triumph was the news that the coach of the U.S. Rifle Team who had come to the range to watch him shoot had said that he was the finest prospect he had ever seen.

There were no triumphs the following semester. At the end of the term the headmaster called Tom and Lydia to his office. He was apologetic, appalled, and baffled. Corky had failed in every subject. In addition, he had become quite belligerent in the classroom. The next morning Lydia took him to Wells, who after a brief examination told her that the boy was passing through a phase. That afternoon he was dropped from the basketball team. One Saturday as he got ready to shoot on the range, the riflery coach put his arm around his shoulders and suggested that he take six months off to get his bearings. Two weeks later he had his first convulsion. Wells immediately called in a neurologist. This one devoted almost half his time to psychiatry. While there is nothing unethical in such medical moonlighting, it is nevertheless a little like being a cobbler and a curator at the same time. The two disciplines have so little in common. The neurologist's diagnosis was a progressive, destructive disease of the central nervous system, cause unknown. The outlook, he felt, was grim.

Soon more ominous signs appeared. Corky began to lose his memory. He became apathetic. He was plagued with choreoathetosis, that combination of jerky and at the same time slow, writhing movements which were not under his control. The time had come, Tom now felt, for a definitive opinion. He took Lydia and his son to the Mayo Clinic in the company jet. There, a high level of measles antibodies was found in the blood and spinal fluid. The neurologist's diagnosis was Dawson's encephalitis, more recently known as subacute sclerosing panencephalitis, or SSPE in doctors' jargon. Not only did the specialist give the Guthries the definitive diagnosis. He explained what it meant.

On rare occasions after a child has apparently recovered from an attack of measles the virus continues to grow undetected in his brain. The incubation period, the symptom-free hiatus, may last for months or even years. Once the disease is detected, death may likewise take months or even years. All the time the measles virus is at work destroying the patient's central nervous system. The disease is one of several, scientists believe, brought on by slow, long-acting viruses which attack the brain and spinal cord. Others, perhaps less well known, are scrapie in cattle and Kuru, prevalent among the primitive Fore people of the Eastern Highlands of New Guinea. This sickness, which once occurred in epidemic form and is still invariably fatal, is caused by a virus, so far unidentified, which takes years to kill its victims. The method of transmission is dependent upon the mourning ritual of the tribe, which consists of the cannibalistic consumption of dead relatives, many of whom are infected with the Kuru virus. Under the pressure of Western civilization, the mourning rites have been abandoned and Kuru is dying out, just as SSPE is disappearing because of the widespread use of measles vaccine. Both conditions are equally devastating. The Mayo Clinic neurologist gave the Guthries a bleak prognosis.

On the way back to New York in the company jet Lydia made no attempt to hide her tears. She held Tom's hand but they did not speak to each other. He did not reproach her for failing to have Corky immunized. She did not mention her negligence. An unspoken agreement made the subject tabu. Corky now stayed at home, cared for by nurses who were on duty around the clock. Within a month his vision began to fail. Two weeks later he was totally blind. Decorticate rigidity, that stiffness of the trunk and limbs which can be produced in experimental animals by the removal of the thinking portion of the brain, set in. Finally he sank into a stupor. The golden boy had changed into what doctors in their bitter moments call a vegetable. Lydia became apathetic and began to lose her looks. When Tom told her that he was going to sell the place in Vermont, she nodded. There was no discussion.

Tom made a final attempt to obtain a more favorable prognosis. Late in November the Guthries took their son to the Children's Medical Center in Boston. There a neurosurgeon performed a biopsy on the frontal lobe of Corky's brain. The tiny piece that he removed was examined under both the electron and the light microscope and placed in tissue culture as well. The immunofluorescent technique showed measles antigen by electron microscopy. And measles virus grew out of the tissue culture. Slides examined under the ordinary light microscope demonstrated extensive destruction of nerve tissue. The Boston pediatricians and neurologists indicated that the prognosis was hopeless.

From time to time during the course of the illness, in fact from the moment he had learned that the slow, long-acting measles virus was devouring Corky's brain, Wells had advised the Guthries against discussing the case with anyone at Adams. He pointed out that since nothing further could be done for the boy, he should be allowed to die in peace, with the family freed from the burden of learned discourses. Talking to the doctors in the hospital about their son's condition could only stimulate them to offer a thousand well-meant suggestions which might open up old wounds in the parents and cause unnecessary physical suffering in the child. As a result of Wells's persuasive arguments, no other medical opinions but his were heard in the Guthries' home. He was the master of the sick room. Lydia was impressed because he never missed his daily house call no matter how busy he was. Tom paid the bills, which amounted to over fifteen hundred dollars a month, and said nothing. Then suddenly early in December the pediatrician asked him in an impressively brief telephone conversation to bring his wife to the office the following day. As soon as he had plundered Keats's laboratory, Wells had decided that Corky would receive the first dose of what he imagined was the virus killer. Certainly no child deserved it more. Besides, his father was rich enough to pay handsomely for it. And to top it all he was a member of the all-powerful seven-man conference committee of the board of trustees.

Seated across the desk from the Guthries in his severely beautiful consultation room, Wells said, "I have just gotten my hands on a small amount, only six doses, of the most powerful solution of interferon yet prepared. I would like Corky to be the first to receive it."

"What is it?" asked Tom. "Something new?"

"It's a virus killer," answered Wells, "and it's as new as tomorrow afternoon's Dow Jones average."

"What effect do you think it will have on Corky?" asked Lydia.

Wells reached the outer limits of expansiveness. "I hope," he replied simply, "that it will cure him."

"Is that possible?" exclaimed Tom.

Wells smiled. "To show you how confident I am, I won't set a fee for my services. I'll handle everything on a contingency basis, just as a lawyer would in a negligence case. If I am not successful,

I won't accept a cent. If I am, well, we will talk about that afterward. I might add that once these six doses are used up, there will be no more in the foreseeable future." He looked thoughtful. "I can't tell you the source of my batch of interferon, but I don't mind confessing that I've been hunting for something like this for Corky ever since we made the diagnosis."

Lydia's cheeks were flushed. "That's the most wonderful news I have ever heard."

"Let's make it front-page news tomorrow," said Wells. "I'm admitting Corky to Adams in the morning."

Lydia had invited old Dr. and Mrs. Guthrie for dinner that night. First everyone drank scotch and water in the drawing room, even Grandma Guthrie, who although she did not approve of alcohol in principle felt that a drop or two would be good for a seventy-four-year-old woman's heart. She listened stony-eyed to her daughter-in-law's report of the new, potent interferon solution and learned that it was going to be administered to Corky in the morning. Then she finished the scotch and soda, the first in the room to do so, and said, "I have to prepare you for the worst, Lydia. That Wells person is a fake."

"I wouldn't put it exactly that way, dear," said her husband. "I've made a few inquiries among the older doctors, and they seem to feel he is merely a low-powered charlatan."

"I don't care what you say," said Lydia. "During the bad times he has been a tower of strength to me."

"Lydia," said the blunt, old doctor, "he's a tower of horse manure."

The following morning at eight o'clock Corky, accompanied by his parents, was admitted to a corner private room on the pediatric floor. At ten thirty Wells, handsome as a young doctor on a television medical serial, and with fourteen residents trailing behind him, walked to the bedside. Lydia rose, awed by his entourage. Tom rose too, but a little more slowly. A trustee as well as a father, he knew who was paying the salaries.

"Dr. Wells," he asked, "how soon do you estimate it will be before the interferon takes effect?"

Thinking back to Keats's experiences with the medication, Wells answered, "Just a few hours, I hope. Would you and Mrs. Guthrie mind stepping outside for a moment?"

As soon as the door closed he started to give a short talk on interferon to the residents. The night before, in the medical library, he had learned something about it himself. The young doctors showed how restless they were by shifting their positions, coughing, and whispering to each other. They felt that it was improper for them to be forced to stand up for such a speech when there was a small lecture room with comfortable seats on the seventh floor. To their obvious relief Wells, though held up by frequent references to his notes, soon finished.

He handed the chief resident a small bottle with six ml. of a colorless, crystal-clear fluid which he had just taken out of his bag. "I want you to inject two ml. intravenously."

"Wouldn't you prefer to inject such an important drug yourself?" the young man asked graciously.

"*Homage au* chief resident," answered Wells, who did not know how to say "chief resident" in French.

Corky was lying stiff and comatose on the bed, his arms and legs ceaselessly making those involuntary, jerky, writhing movements characteristic of choreoathetosis. Although two nurses held the patient's right arm motionless, the resident had difficulty getting into the vein at the bend of the elbow. He remembered for a fleeting moment what Keats had once told him when he could not be found for an emergency admission.

"A pediatric resident has two functions," Keats had said. "To answer the phone on the first ring and to get into a vein on the first attempt."

The chief resident was not measuring up to the definition. He had to try four times before he was able to inject the solution. As soon as he pulled out the needle, Wells replaced the bottle in his bag, sniffed twice, and walked out. The smell had become pronounced. Corky was incontinent of urine and feces. Already the two nurses were laying down fresh sheets.

Wells went to the central station and wrote in the chart for an hour. Not for nothing was he called the father of Adams' paper pediatric service. After he had placed the reports from the Mayo Clinic and the Boston Children's Medical Center in their proper places he returned to the room. Tom and Lydia were staring glumly at their son. His condition was the same. Indeed, it would have been surprising if it had been anything else. Two ml., which was less than one-half teaspoonful, of ordinary salt solution had never affected a twelve-year-old boy for better or for worse. Not a member of the house staff was in the room. They could have been found, except during lunch hour, attending lectures and seminars on the comfortable seats of the conference rooms until two thirty. Then they would go to one of the many clinics in the outpatient department, where they were permitted to examine patients in the main unsupervised, or else to sit and talk to each other if there was nothing else to do. At four they went to the pediatric floor for sign-out rounds, a brief ceremony which gave them the right to return to wife or husband depending on which sex they were, a determination occasionally not easily made especially from the rear. The residents were not yet unionized. Nevertheless, a combination of Gompers, Reuther, and Meany, backed by Bridges, Shanker, and DiLourie could hardly have improved upon their contract. These as yet medical amateurs received fourteen to eighteen thousand dollars a year with a fine room thrown in for a forty-hour week most of which was devoted to their education.

Wells went to his office for his morning appointments. When he returned at two in the afternoon he found his patient's condition unchanged. The decision he arrived at was a painful one. It would be necessary, he felt, to use the remainder of the solution he had brought with him. So disturbed was he that he forgot to ask the Guthries to leave. It took him ten minutes to find a vein and stay in it. He had not done any intravenous work since his residency at the Medical Center. To the Guthries, who had observed the procedure in uncomfortable silence, he explained that this time he had injected a double dose of the priceless material. When he returned at five thirty, Corky was no better.

He looked at the Guthries and said, "I feel as bad about this as you do."

Interestingly enough, he was quite sincere. Had he not thrown away thirty-five thousand dollars? Of course, he had never had a son.

At seven o'clock that night Lydia and Tom left the hospital for their home, where the senior Dr. and Mrs. Guthrie were awaiting the news. When Tom finished his report, Grandma Guthrie said,

"If you pay that man a penny, you are not the financial genius people say you are."

"I may not be a financial genius," said Tom, "but I am my mother's son. He won't get a cent. That was the deal."

Old Dr. Guthrie was muttering to himself.

"What did you say, dear?" asked his wife.

"A tower of horse manure," muttered the old man.

At eight the next morning Tom knocked on the open door of Trudy Starr's office and walked in. She rose at once. After motioning her to her chair behind the desk, he sat down himself and said,

"I suppose I am taking advantage of my position as a trustee by barging in here like this, but I need your advice. I simply must have a woman's point of view. My wife is in bed crying. She's been crying on and off all night. We never expected to have a child and when this golden boy was born, we expected everything." He shook his head. "It's the disappointment that's pushed her to the edge. Wells really sold her a bill of goods. What I'd like to know from you is this: Should I take Corky home right now or should I let him stay here a couple of months until she can learn to live with despair? You're not full, are you?"

Trudy stood up, closed the door, and sat down again.

"You know, Miss Starr," said Tom, "the trustees consider you one of the crown jewels of Adams."

Trudy gave him a pleasant smile. "Then I'm going to take advantage of my position, too. I don't think you should do either. And I don't think you should succumb to despair. Dr. Keats, the senior man in the Department of Pediatrics, and in my opinion, number one in everything, really has a minute amount of a genuine virus killer. I have been on staff of two of the finest hospitals abroad, and I'm not easily impressed, but this drug is simply miraculous. A little while ago I saw him inject it into a boy of Corky's age who also was dying of a rare disease of the nervous system. All his muscles, including those he breathed with, were paralyzed. A few hours after the injection he was completely well." She put her elbows on the desk and leaned toward Guthrie. "Why don't you take your wife to see Dr. Keats tomorrow. He's an honest man."

"You're very kind. I will. A second disappointment should not be as bad as the first. Besides, my Scotch Presbyterian mother has always insisted that there is a God."

He looked around him at the bare walls of the austere office and said, "Won't you let me give you a picture?"

Trudy, thinking of her collection at home, which by now was worth over half a million dollars, started to laugh. "Please! I already have a picture."

Tom studied the big, beautiful, blonde woman who radiated health, strength, and efficiency, and decided that there was hope.

The next morning he and Lydia, accompanied by Grandma Guthrie, who had insisted on coming, seated themselves in front of Keats's desk.

"Doctor," said Tom, "Miss Starr said that you had a small amount of a very potent virus killer."

"She told me," said Jim.

"I hope I won't have to repeat the long story of what happened to Corky. I'm afraid it would upset my wife."

"I'm familiar with the case," said Jim.

Suddenly Lydia felt that this huge man with the bent nose and the hard eyes was going to give her the courage to break the tabu.

"Doctor, it's all my fault, you know. Everything that's happened to Corky is my fault. His living death is my fault. I had ten years in which to have him immunized against measles, but I didn't. I was too busy with other things."

"This disease is so rare," said Jim, "that most doctors have never seen a case. Thousands of children must get measles before one comes down with Dawson's encephalitis. What happened to Corky was not an example of negligence. It was an act of fate. But more important is the fact that the vaccine is only ninety-six percent effective. He could have received it and still have come down with measles. Now what do you say to that?"

"Is that really true?" said Lydia. Tears were streaming down her face but she was smiling. "Are those really the facts?"

Keats put his hands on the desk and leaned forward. His tremendous shoulders and tough face made him look especially formidable. "Madam, do I look like one of those kids who just graduated from medical school?"

"No, no! Of course not, Doctor," said Tom.

Color was coming to Lydia's cheeks. She was beginning to look like the girl he had married.

"Oh, I wouldn't say that, dear," she said. "If the doctor had a little more hair, he might at that."

The three Guthries hazarded a smile.

Tom looked Jim in the eye. "Could you spare a little of the virus killer for my boy?"

"Certainly, if Dr. Wells has no objection."

"I asked him to step down a few minutes ago. Will you do it now? Will you take care of Corky?"

Jim nodded.

"Do you really think it will help him?" asked Lydia.

There was a long silence. "I'm certain that it will neutralize the slow-acting measles virus that is in his central nervous system," said Jim. "But that's only part of the problem. Most of his brain has already been destroyed. It's like calling in the firemen after the building has burnt almost to the ground. They can put out the flames, but can they rebuild the house?"

"Will you try, Doctor?" asked Grandma Guthrie. "He used to be such a handsome boy."

Jim wheeled on her. "And why shouldn't he have been, with your genes in his body!"

Grandma Guthrie smiled. At that moment she reminded Tom of the mother he had known when he was going to college.

Jim rose. As he ushered the Guthries to the door he said, "I'll inject Corky at eight tomorrow morning."

Suddenly Lydia turned, stood on her toes, and kissed him.

"Ah!" exclaimed Grandma Guthrie, "if only I were thirty years younger!"

As the Guthries walked toward the car she said, "That man is all wool and a yard wide."

"He's a yard wide all right," said her son.

After instructing his secretary to call Wells's nurse and tell her that he was taking over the case, Jim went to Adams and read through Corky's chart. Then, assisted by Trudy, he examined him thoroughly. The two special-duty nurses, who at a signal from their superior had hurried to the other end of the room, were astounded to see the legendary Miss Starr, the supervisor, the administrator, the graduate student, helping a doctor perform a routine task.

"Do you think there is something between them?" one of them whispered.

The other, an old spinster, beamed. "I hope so."

When Tom and Lydia walked into their son's hospital room promptly at eight the next morning, Jim was carefully removing two ml. of the virus killer from the six in the bottle Trudy held before him. Although Corky's jerky and squirming movements were particularly violent, Jim entered the vein at the bend of the elbow with ease and injected the contents of the syringe in a few seconds. Tom was impressed. Nothing happened for a half an hour. Then Jim noticed that the choreoathetotic movements were lessening. In another half hour they had ceased entirely. The boy appeared to be in a deep sleep. One hour after this he was making perfectly coordinated movements of the upper and lower extremities. The terrible stiffness of the trunk, neck, arms, and legs had disappeared. Jim performed a complete physical examination for the second time. Now it was normal. In spite of the rapid improvement, he looked worried. The Guthries sat speechless. The silence was becoming oppressive. Suddenly Corky raised his head and cried, "Mother!"

Lydia hurried to the bed and put her hand on her son's cheek. "I'm here, Corky."

"Mother, I don't remember anything. I can't see. Why can't I see?"

"Because you've been very sick, dear."

"Won't I ever be able to see, Mother?"

Lydia raised her arms in supplication to the huge man with the troubled eyes as if she beheld in him Christ returned to earth.

"Be patient, Corky," said Jim, but he was looking at Lydia.

He walked to the table, took a sterile syringe, and removed another ml. of the virus killer from the bottle Trudy held up to him. Without a word he injected the solution into the vein so quickly that Corky hardly felt the needle prick. After ten minutes he flashed a light from his ophthalmoscope into the boy's eyes. The pupils reacted at once.

"Did you see anything?" asked Jim.

"A light," answered the boy.

Jim waited fifteen minutes more. Then he passed his hand before his patient's eyes. "Did you see anything this time?"

"Something moving."

Jim laid a towel over Corky's eyes and sat on the bed. The Guthries did not dare to say a word. After an hour Jim removed the towel. Nothing happened. Suddenly Corky sat up and screamed, "I can see!"

He stared at Jim. "Are you the doctor?"

Jim nodded.

"Wow!" said the boy. "You're big and mean-looking." Then he remembered his manners. "I don't mean you're ugly or anything like that. It's just that you're not handsome like my father."

Trudy put her hand on Jim's shoulder. "Pay no attention to him. He is just repeating the opinions he's heard at home."

Corky was in his mother's arms. It took a long time for her to release him. When at last she did, Tom walked to the bed and shook his son's hand.

"Where's Grandma, Dad?"

"She's home praying for you," replied his father.

"Corky," said Jim, "get up and run around the room."

The boy obeyed. Jim regarded him critically. A born athlete, he decided. Suddenly Corky stopped and looked at him.

"I remember. The coach dropped me from the rifle team. Do you think I'll ever be able to shoot again?"

"We'll see," said Jim and walked out of the room.

The cold December wind lashed his face as he tramped through the streets. He had no muffler so he turned up his overcoat collar and hunched his shoulders. In the fourth store he found what he was looking for. When he returned to his patient's room he was carrying a large cardboard box. He opened it and tacked a dart board to the wall.

"Corky, step over to the other side of the room. Miss Starr once lived in England. She'll show you how to hold these things."

He handed Trudy the darts. She demonstrated the grip.

"Do I get a practice shot?" asked the boy.

"Nope," said Jim.

Three times Corky raised his arm and threw. Three times a dart hit the bull's-eye.

"You'll shoot," said Jim and walked out.

One hour later Corky was home. Since no one expected him, the celebration was impromptu. After dinner that night the cook, followed by the two maids and the window-cleaning man, a great family favorite, carried in a three-tiered birthday cake. Everyone sang "Happy Birthday" even though Corky had been born in June.

"There are no candles on the cake," said Tom to his son, "because you were just born, a second time and at twelve years of age."

Corky cut the cake. His hand was as steady as a surgeon's. Only then was the champagne served. Everyone including the boy and the servants had to accept a full glass whether they liked champagne or not.

Corky raised his glass. "To Keats. He's gotta be the greatest doctor in the world."

"He's more than a great doctor," said his grandmother. "He's a man. A very attractive man." She leaned over and kissed her seventy-seven-year-old husband on the lips. "The second I've managed to find in a long lifetime."

After a few moments Corky went upstairs to watch television.

Grandma Guthrie turned her shrewd Scotch face to her son. "Remember what I taught you. After a great success, always give to a good cause." She smiled. "A doctor can be a good cause."

"Especially," said old Dr. Guthrie, "if he's worked at Adams for thirty years and never made a nickel."

"If Tom doesn't listen to you," said Lydia, "he'll listen to me. Unless he sends Dr. Keats a princely fee, I'll never go to bed with him again, or at least until I can't hold out anymore, which is usually about a week."

Tom and the old doctor froze. But Grandma Guthrie was not shocked. She smiled and said,

"I still think my system is the best, twice a week, rain or shine, winter and summer."

Old Dr. Guthrie took a slim datebook from his pocket and leafed through its pages until he found the place. "You're absolutely right, dear," he said as he rose. "It's time we left."

Three days later Tom Guthrie telephoned Jim during his office hours. "The reason we haven't called you sooner is that Corky has been so well. My wife insisted on having him tested by a psychologist. His I.Q. is still a hundred seventy, just as if his intelligence had been developing during his illness. By the way, what about your bill?"

"Oh, I don't know," said Jim. He sounded embarrassed. "Anything you want." Suddenly his voice brightened. "Maybe a small contribution to the Department of Pediatrics."

The investment banker laughed so hard that he began to cough. During a particularly severe paroxysm he hung up.

An hour and a half later a messenger left two envelopes with Jim's secretary. The one on top was labeled number one, the other, written in red ink, number two. Jim opened number one. It was addressed to Dr. James Keats, The World's Worst Businessman, and read,

"Since you were unwise enough to allow me to set the fee, I am sending you the enclosed check in complete payment for all services rendered to date to me and my family, including the care and treatment of my son in John Quincy Adams Hospital."

The check was for one thousand dollars.

The second letter was addressed to Dr. James Keats and read,

"It is important that you realize that the enclosed is not in payment of a fee. You have already been paid. It is a gift from my wife and me to express our admiration and affection for you as a man and as a doctor. Since I am going to pay all gift taxes, my accountant and my tax lawyer both assure me that you do not have to declare this as income next April fifteenth. My wife and I send our gratitude; my mother, her love."

It was signed "Tom and Lydia." Clipped to the letter was a check for twenty-five thousand dollars.

Jim smiled. For the first time in his life he was going to have money in the bank. The telephone rang. He did not hear it. His secretary walked in and touched his shoulder.

"Professor Choate," she said.

He picked up the receiver.

"Jim, I have bad news for you," said Choate. "We couldn't get anywhere with your virus killer. We tried everything in the book, animal injection, tissue culture, radio immuno assay, chemical analysis. Not a clue. You know, Jim, we really had so little to work with. How much do you have left?"

"One dose," answered Jim.

14

ALTHOUGH TRUDY STARR was not required to report for duty until eight in the morning, she had recently taken to arriving at her office fifteen minutes earlier ever since she realized that Jim came to visit her regularly at this time. Often he brought a few flowers for her desk; the day before Thanksgiving, an orchid. This blustery December morning as they sat facing each other, she asked,

"What are you going to do about your wife?"

"Divorce her."

"When?"

"As soon as they appoint a new director of Pediatrics. I don't want to rock the boat now."

Trudy looked at her beautifully kept hands. "Does she suspect that you know about her affair with Wells?"

Jim shook his head.

She laughed. "I can just see both of you at home. You must act like two unarmed soldiers, a German and an Englishman, crouching in the same foxhole during a bombardment in World War II and trying to ignore each other's uniforms."

He shrugged. "We haven't had anything to do with each other for a long time. I haven't slept with her in three years. Or anyone else for that matter. I'm afraid I've lost the knack." He paused. "She speaks to me occasionally, only now she is a little more civil."

"And after the divorce?"

He smiled. "I'd like to go steady with you."

Trudy laughed. "Do I at least get your fraternity pin?" She shook her head. "Jimmy, I don't know what to do with you. Anyway, it's a beginning."

"Toward an unconsummated marriage with an impotent wreck of fifty-four? I wouldn't let you. For me, marriage with you will always remain an impossible dream."

"For a scientist you have been very unscientific during the past three years. You haven't tested your potency. All it needs is a little exercise. And as for that impossible dream, if you were Sir Galahad and someone tossed the Holy Grail into your lap, you would still insist that it was an impossible dream." She looked away for a moment. "I think you ought to tell the medical board that Wells stole the virus killer or what he thought was the virus killer. And I think you should do it right away."

"I suppose you're right but it goes against the grain."

"You will have to do it if you want that job. For an honest man politics means doing things that go against the grain. Don't be so passive, Jimmy dear. Get mean. Make believe you're playing football for Columbia again. When does the medical board meet?"

"Later this month. That's when they're supposed to elect a new director. Their nomination goes to the joint conference committee."

"What in the world is that?"

"It consists of the seven directors and the seven most important trustees. The seven trustees pump the doctors, and later, when they meet alone, come up with the decision. The full thirty-man board always ratifies their choice."

"Is Mr. Guthrie one of the seven?" asked Trudy.

"Yes, and very powerful."

"Promise me one thing, Jimmy, that you will spill the beans before that seven-man trustees' committee makes up its mind."

"I promise." He stood up as if with difficulty. "I'm sore from the kick in the pants you just gave me."

"I'm not worried. Worse things have happened to you on the football field."

Jim walked to the group of four automatic elevators and pressed the button. Nothing happened. Because of their unpredictability and infrequent appearances he habitually referred to them as the vertical Long Island Railroad. If Hexter, the administrator, ran them as efficiently as he balanced the budget, he reflected, nobody would ever be kept waiting. A little old lady, obviously tense and nervous, was walking up and down near him. He looked at his wristwatch and said,

"Madam, the next elevator arrives at eight-o-six."

She smiled and looked at her wristwatch, too. To Jim's amazement, promptly at eight-o-six one of the doors opened. Clustered in the center of the car were two residents, a middle-aged woman, and a surgical consultant in his early seventies. In the corner, as if keeping himself apart, was a tall, elegant young doctor with the face of an El Greco grandee. Everyone watched Jim help the little old lady across the threshold. As soon as the door opened on the third floor, the surgeon inclined his head toward the middle-aged woman, who smiled and started to walk out. But she was not fast enough. One of the residents slid past her, shoving her slightly to the side and made his way toward the cafeteria. As soon as the woman and the consultant recovered from their surprise, they left too, turning toward the X-ray section on the right. When the elevator reached the ground floor Jim made a courtly bow to the little old lady, extended his arm palm upward, and said, "Please!" Suddenly he felt the resident behind him trying to shoulder his way forward. He nudged the youngster gently with his hip, swung around, and with knees bent, planted himself directly in his path. The member of the house staff took a step to the side in an effort to get to the door but soon discovered what the linesmen in the Ivy League had learned thirty-five years before—that Keats was a hard man to get past when he was protecting a teammate. The little old lady patted her defender on the shoulder, said, "Thank you," and was gone. Jim, who had been smiling grimly, now laughed, turned around, and walked out.

What had that boy just learned, he asked himself? Nothing, he decided, absolutely nothing, except, perhaps, always to sneak ahead of an old lady but let a big guy go first. Inside an elevator the members of the house staff ignored age, rank, preeminence, sex, disability, and infirmity. Outside an elevator they were not much better. He thought of complaining to Hexter about their mass discourtesy but shied away from the idea when he realized that thermal underwear was de rigeur when confronting that chilling personality on a winter's day. And the complaint department which the administrator had created a few years earlier although run with great efficiency could do nothing in this case.

The bureau had begun as an offshoot of his unsuccessful attempt to fire Oldham, a sixty-three-year-old assistant who had worked at Adams for three and a half decades. Hexter had as little use for an employee over sixty as for an automobile that had run over sixty thousand miles. The trustees felt differently. They would not permit him to cashier the old retainer. Since he could not get rid of his subordinate, he decided to utilize his assets, the leonine face, white wavy mane, and sonorous basso voice. For a week he coached Oldham on how to perform his new duties. Then he installed him in an imposing office with luxurious chairs and a massive desk which he was instructed to keep bare except for the red telephone in the center. Soon people began to stream in. Oldham would listen attentively to the members of a patient's family, nodding occasionally over tented fingers and showing by his expression that he understood their grievances. Perhaps what emerged was a resident's error. When all the accusations had been aired, the old man would lift the red telephone and dial the floor where the culprit was to be found. "Too busy to come to the phone? Doing something really important?" he would mimic, holding the mouthpiece a little away from him with obvious distaste. "Nothing is as important as satisfying a patient's family. I want him on the line within sixty seconds," he would roar. Then he would drum on the empty desk with his fingers and thumb while the members of the family surreptitiously consulted their wristwatches. And just as they had expected, within the minute they would hear him say, "Doctor, grave charges have been brought against you." They were proud of themselves as they listened to the raw and rambling facts which they had just provided become transformed into convincing and eloquent arguments in the mouth of this formidable prosecutor. But the long silence which followed impressed them even more. The assistant administrator, they could see, was not only formidable but fair. The accused certainly had the right to be heard. At last Oldham's lips would curl and he would say, "Good, Doctor, very good, but not good enough." Then he would denounce his prey in terms so savage, so biting, and so merciless that they would become embarrassed. They had never believed that a day would come when they would hear anyone talk this way to a doctor, especially one as important as a resident. As soon as Oldham hung up he would rise, his silver hair even whiter as a result of the ordeal, extend his big, fleshy hand, and say to them, "All of us at John Quincy Adams Hospital ask you to accept our collective apology." Here he would smile knowingly and add, "I think it unlikely that this incident will ever be repeated."

The next group might consist of a mother, father, and grandmother come to complain because their little girl had lain in feces and urine for an hour in spite of their repeated efforts to persuade a nurse to change the sheets. Oldham would listen attentively, shaking his head from time to time and murmuring, "Imagine, a little child!" Again he would lift the red telephone. Again he would ask to speak to the accused. "And why can't she come to the telephone?" he would demand. "The call of nature?" Here he would raise his head and sit even straighter. "When I am on duty, I never listen to the call of nature." Again he would give the sixty-second ultimatum. Again the terrible drumbeat would issue from the desk. The horrified relatives could envision the nurse hurrying clumsily in the toilet. But no, why should they feel guilty, they would ask themselves, especially after what she had done to their little girl? Again would come the clever presentation of their case, the period of fair-minded judgment, and the savage denunciation, this time ending cruelly with, "Miss, I have serious doubts about your ability to ever assume the responsibilities of motherhood." At last, at the very end, the moving apology.

Hundreds of angry complainants had rushed into that office. Everyone had left satisfied, serene, and avenged. The reason why Hexter's system worked so well was that the red telephone had never been connected.

Walking along the main corridor, Jim decided that it would be useless to complain. The house staff's attitudes would never change until the world's did. You started off pushing little old ladies to one side; you ended up dropping bombs on little old countries like Vietnam. The elegant young doctor who had held himself apart in the corner of the elevator caught up with him, saluted, and said in almost flawless English with a mere trace of a Spanish accent,

"Two ears and the tail!"

They both stopped. Jim smiled and said, "Aren't you one of the first-year pediatric residents?"

"I am, sir. My name is José Cheecheecastanango."

"I remember it well."

A hospital has background music just as a movie does, Jim said to himself. In Adams it was the continuous monotone of humdrum names which came over the public address system, "Dr. Brown, Dr. Taylor, Dr. Kelly, Dr. Horowitz, Dr. Schultz, Dr. Long, Dr. Levy," followed by a brief, merciful silence. Then, at last, the page operator would call out in the sexy voice she had been saving for just this moment, "Dr. José Cheecheecastanango!" And suddenly every nurse in the place, he was sure, would hear castanets, the staccato of Flamenco dancing, and Alicia de la Rocha playing de Falle's "Nights in the Gardens of Spain."

"How do you like it at Adams?" Jim asked.

"Not much. I applied to the Medical Center, but Dr. Locke sent me here." He laughed, and his black El Greco eyes flashed. "When he found out about my family, though, he telephoned me and told me to come to the Medical Center for the last two years of my residency."

"What's this with your family?"

"They are very rich, very distinguished, and very liberal—or as liberal as you can be in Argentina and still stay out of jail. And they have been there a long time, sir. Governments come and governments go, but Swiss bank accounts go on forever."

"Why don't you like it here?" asked Jim.

"Dr. Dummer is a foolish old man. And Dr. Wells." He shrugged. "Will you be offended if I use an American expression?"

"Of course not."

"Dr. Wells," continued José, "is as deep as pee on a hot rock in the sun."

"But considerably more attractive to women," said Jim. "Are you married?"

"No, sir. I won't marry until I am a doctor and a man."

"When do you think that will be?"

"When I finish my residency, when I am no longer being paid to learn. Until then I will have to resort to fornication and birth control and pray that God will be more permissive than the Church."

Jim nodded. "He probably is. Sometimes the army is more militant than the king. But you still haven't told me specifically why you think so little of the Department of Pediatrics."

"Well, sir, there are at present fourteen medical pediatric patients on the service, most of them semiprivate and under the care of their own doctors. To look after these fourteen children there are fourteen residents. Each of us is assigned one patient. That is our case load. We are not encouraged to familiarize ourselves with the patients of the other residents. Occasionally we are sent to the nursery, but the infants there are mostly normal newborns. And once in a while we go to the emergency room. It's nothing like the emergency rooms on television. Adams is not in a ghetto neighborhood. There is just enough work to keep us occupied for maybe an hour or two a day. The rest of the time is taken up with lectures, talks, demonstrations, conferences, seminars, and clinics where unfortunately we do not learn very much. For this I get fourteen thousand dollars a year, I who just got out of medical school six months ago. I am being paid to go to lectures. My conscience is beginning to hurt. I would give the money back, but then I would be accused of being a South American millionaire who was spoiling a wonderful racket for everybody else."

"What about rounds?"

"They are made almost exclusively by Dr. Dummer. Once, when he was young, his rounds may have been mediocre. Now they are simply bad. I know that there are fine pediatricians among the older attendings, but they are permitted to make rounds only once a month. And they are never allowed to make rounds with Dr. Dummer. Evidently he couldn't stand the competition. But as you say in this country, for us residents the fringe benefits are excellent. Dr. Wells, whom Dr. Dummer has put in charge of us, sends us to meetings and conventions all over the world at the hospital's expense. He tells me that I can go to the Argentine whenever I please. The only trouble is that I just came from there."

"You have managed to take in a lot in six months," said Jim.

"That is true. All the same, I feel like the aficionado who came to Madrid in the old days for the bullfights but never saw Juan Belmonte."

"I don't get you."

"I missed seeing your performances with Charlie Prince and Corky Guthrie. In parts of my country you would have either been put up for canonization or burnt at the stake."

Jim smiled. "I'll call you if I ever do anything like that again."

José bowed. "I hope you are the next director of Pediatrics, sir. For all our sakes."

Jim went to the doctors' lounge. He saw that Scotti was signing in.

"Old football buddy," said the Director of Medicine, "could we talk?"

They sat down on a small couch in the corner.

"I hear you've got hold of a virus killer that makes you Red Grange, O. J. Simpson, Larry Czsonka, and Hippocrates rolled into one," said Scotti. "What is it? Level with the man who used to open up those big holes for you in the old days."

"I have no idea what it is. You remember Bill Choate from medical school, don't you?"

"Sure, big Nobel brain, no brawn, good raconteur."

"Right. I got the stuff from him," said Jim.

He told the Director of Medicine the story of the virus killer.

"How do you think it works?" asked Scotti.

"First, it destroys the virus that's in the patient's body," said Jim. "Second, it restores the tissues to the state they were in before the virus struck, in other words back to normal."

"You used it on Tom Guthrie's son, didn't you, after Wells made an ass of himself by promising to cure the boy?"

"Yes, but I'd rather not talk about it now. All he injected was ordinary isotonic saline solution."

Scotti's eyes widened. "I'll bring that up at the meeting next Wednesday afternoon. Not that it will do any good."

"Do you think Wells will get the job?" asked Jim.

"Oh, no. But the medical board won't vote you in either. What I'm afraid of is that the trustees may insist that we get someone from the outside, someone like Wells. We didn't look very hard this time. After the meeting we may have to."

"The directors are all former Adams residents, aren't they?" asked Jim.

"Sure," said Scotti. "No matter how much we fight, we're still alumni. It's the Horatio Alger story, up from the ranks. But things are changing fast. Throughout the country the search is on for new blood. A man may work his heart out for a hospital for twenty years. Then, just as he attains the maturity to make a good chief, a youngster is called in from another institution and given the job over his head. If the kid is pleasant and stays out of trouble, the hospital may be stuck with him for thirty years no matter how mediocre he is."

"If Adams can't develop men for its top jobs anymore, it's not the hospital we once knew," said Jim.

"True," said Scotti, "but that's not why I wanted to talk to you." He gave Jim a penetrating stare. "Have you thought of using your virus killer against cancer?"

"Yes, and I rejected the idea."

"Why? The Rous sarcoma in chickens is caused by a virus. There may be some connection between carcinoma of the cervix and the herpes virus. And there are reputable investigators who believe that viruses may play a part in the development of leukemia."

"But there is no definite proof that they cause cancer in humans. Why all this sudden interest in a cure for cancer, anyway?"

"Because Frank Ray is dying of an inoperable carcinoma of the lung. If there is one chance in a thousand that the virus killer might help him, I think you ought to let him have it."

"Okay, I will, but it won't work."

"Will you talk to him about it soon?"

"Of course."

"When?"

"Right now," said Jim.

They both stood up. Scotti patted his friend on the back.

"Old Forty-one. Always good for five yards."

Jim took the elevator to the third floor, turned right, and walked to Frank Ray's office. Guarding the door while she typed with phenomenal speed was his private secretary, Jenny Velvet. She was in her late twenties, blonde, beautiful, and creamy, a Miss Vanilla Milkshake. On her lovely face there were no lines either of strain or excessive intelligence. To Jim she looked as if she had just stepped out of her bath. He meant it not in the cliché sense that indicated cleanliness, but in the carnal sense that implied that she was revealing her body to him for the first time, an effect her tight-fitting black dress did nothing to diminish. He was sure she made the same impression when she wore a fur coat. It seemed hard to believe, he mused, that such divine beauty walked out of a tub every morning in a twelve-story apartment house on Second Avenue. More likely it was that she breasted the foamy waves off the coast of Cythera like Aphrodite Anadyomene, and then was wafted to the streets of Manhattan miraculously clothed. And she had this in common with the laughter-loving goddess. She never used perfume. Her own faint, natural scent of musk was a more potent aphrodisiac than anything Chanel or Houbigant had yet manufactured. Mrs. Velvet said of her daughter that she had more gentlemen friends than she knew what to do with, forgetting that they were neither gentlemen nor friends. Jenny's swains were oafs. Often while stroking her in precoital play one of them would say, to show that he had a way with words as well as with women, "Sweetie, your skin feels like velvet." To which she would invariably reply in a high-pitched, irritable voice, "What did you expect it to feel like, a nail file?" Ah, Jenny was one for repartee, her admirers would boast. Actually she knew very little about anything except typing and stenography and sex. She was in effect an idiot savant, like those adolescents who could not get through grade school but were masters at chess. But she was a ravishing idiot savant and a connoisseur of eroticism. Jim she held in high esteem because he was so big and mean-looking.

She gave him one of her wide-open "I'm a woman, you're a man—what are we waiting for, you fool?" smiles, and without finding out whether her boss was busy, said with a jerk of her thumb, "Go right in."

Jim knocked, walked into the tiny office, and closed the door. Ray, who was seated behind his desk scanning a report, stopped coughing and said,

"Excuse me. Sit down." He smiled. "Miss Velvet likes you, Jim, otherwise she would never have let you in like this. She says you are the most virile man in Adams."

If she only knew, said Jim to himself sadly.

"If you've come about the directorship," continued Ray, "all I know is that John and I will vote for you. The fearsome foursome—Dummer, Grant, Bligh, and Akt—will vote for Wells. That leaves Airov. I have a hunch he will vote with us. If he does, the score will be four to three in favor of Wells, a result the trustees will regard as a deadlock. After that nobody knows what will happen." He gave Jim a shrewd look. "Tom Guthrie is very powerful. He's a friend of the chairman of the board."

"Thank you, Frank, I'm grateful. But I didn't come here to talk about the directorship. I came here to talk to you about a virus killer." He repeated what he had just told Scotti. "John and I think," he added, "that it might be worth a try against that chronic pulmonary infection of yours."

"Chronic pulmonary infection!" echoed Ray derisively. "You know damn well that I have an inoperable carcinoma of the lung. Show me one piece of incontrovertible evidence that proves that CA of the lung is caused by a virus. It's simplistic nonsense to think that all you have to do is kill a virus and the cancer patient will live happily ever after. What about the unlimited cell proliferation, the complex immune processes, the modifications of DNA and RNA, the unknown enzymes, the point of no return?"

"What harm can it do, Frank? A little of the stuff can't hurt you."

"Do you think I am worried about it hurting me? How much do you have left?"

"Quite a bit," said Jim.

"Come on, tell me exactly how much."

"Three ml."

"How many doses is that?"

Jim hesitated. "One dose," he said at last.

Ray looked down at his feet. "You know, Jim, dying is hard. And toward the end there are not many things to hold on to. I've got one, a relatively clear conscience." He looked up. "I'm not going to let anyone take that away from me, not even you and John. If I am destined to die of a pulmonary hemorrhage, if I am going to drown in my own blood, I don't want to feel when I hear the big roar that I deprived a child of life, the life you could have saved with the last dose of the virus killer."

He had a violent paroxysm of coughing. When he removed the handkerchief from his mouth, he stood up and said,

"Excuse me for being so rough with you. But a man has to act rough when he turns down an offer like yours. I'm grateful, more grateful than I would care to explain to you." A smile lit up his gaunt face. "You may pat Miss Velvet on her behind when you leave."

Jim shook his head. "I'd rather not start something I couldn't finish."

For the first time Ray seemed a little crestfallen. "She will be so disappointed." Suddenly he brightened. "You don't mind if she pats you on your behind, do you?"

"Not at all," said Jim, always the gentleman.

Ray opened the door and nodded to Miss Velvet. On the way out Jim passed close to her desk. She continued to type rapidly with one hand while patting him gently on the buttocks with the other.

As he walked toward the elevator, he peered into the rooms on both sides of the corridor. The X-ray machines looked so big, and Frank Ray had seemed so little. He must have lost fifty pounds.

15

AT PRECISELY four P.M. Wednesday the twenty-sixth of December 1973, Courtney Akt called the meeting of the medical board to order. He sat rather pointedly on the same side of the table as Dummer, Bligh, and Grant, directly opposite their opponents, Scotti and Ray. Far away at one end, as if to indicate by his isolation that he belonged to neither party, was Airov. At the other, Hexter, the administrator, occupied a straight-backed chair.

Akt tapped on the table with his ballpoint pen. "This meeting may be the most important we have held in years. Today we take the first step, and it will be a big one, toward replacing Dr. Dummer as Director of Pediatrics." He smiled. "Not that anyone can ever take Evan's place."

Hexter frowned at what he considered unnecessary sentimentality. "I have some news not unrelated to the raison d'être of this meeting. Mr. Guthrie has just given two hundred and fifty thousand dollars toward the creation of a department of pediatric virology. By this time we should all know why. Mr. Crunch, the chairman of the board of trustees, has matched his friend's contribution. An additional half million will have to be raised, preferably in the next six months. That's when the building which will house this department will be completed. Running the latest addition to Adams will be the responsibility of the director of Pediatrics. You can see how important this news makes your decision today."

"Do you mean to tell me," said Grant, "that a department of virology will not be the responsibility of the Director of Laboratories?" An artery in his forehead was pulsing.

Hexter gave him a wintry smile. "I mean to tell you just that." He turned to the entire board. "It will be called the Corky Guthrie and Clair Crunch Department of Pediatric Virology."

"Is Clair the chairman's wife or his mother?" asked Bligh, trying

183

to show by his wrinkled-nose, supercilious expression that he was not really curious, merely polite.

"Neither," answered Hexter. "She is his eleven-year-old daughter. He hopes that she will grow up to be the protector, benefactor, and patron saint of the new department."

"A relationship something like that between Mrs. Payson and the New York Mets," said Scotti. "Maybe later on Corky will marry Clair and the division will be renamed the Corky and Clair Guthrie Department of Pediatric Virology. That will make everything easier and take up less space on the sign."

"May I remind you, Dr. Scotti," said Hexter, "that this is a serious matter."

"So is marriage," replied Scotti.

"Let's get on with the meeting," said Akt irritably. "Will the secretary please read the minutes?"

Presented gravely and in great detail by Grant, they were adopted in a rumble of ayes.

"Committee reports," said Akt tersely.

They were given in abbreviated form by the directors.

"New business," announced the president of the medical board.

"Caries" Grant lifted eight monographs bound in blue plastic, dropped one on the table in front of him, and passed the others to his fellow directors and Hexter. Imprinted in gold on each booklet were the words "Constitution and By-Laws of the John Quincy Adams Hospital."

"If you will turn to page eighteen, two lines from the bottom," said Grant, "you will see a sentence which starts, 'If any member of the medical staff is continually absent for over three months, he shall . . .' Now 'continual' means over and over again. 'Continuous' means unbroken. The correct word here is 'continuously.'"

"You know that any change in the constitution and by-laws has to be approved by the joint conference committee and the board of trustees," warned Akt.

"I know that," said Grant.

"Make the motion," said Akt wearily.

"I move that 'continuously' be substituted for 'continually' on page eighteen of the constitution and by-laws."

"Discussion," said Akt.

Nobody said anything.

"All those in favor say aye," intoned Akt.

There were a few grunts.

"Contrary-minded," said Akt.

One director belched. The belch was not counted as a vote against the motion.

"If you will turn to page twenty-seven, fourteen lines from the top," continued Grant, "you will see a sentence which begins, 'If any member of the professional staff shall discover a new drug, he shall be required to . . .' Now you can only discover a thing if it is already in existence. Columbus discovered America, for example. You can't discover a *new* drug. The sentence should read, 'invent a new drug.' "

"Make the motion," said Akt. He sounded quite tired.

It was quickly passed.

Grant rustled his copy of the constitution. "Turning to page thirty-six, two lines from the top, you will see, 'If in official correspondence the sender of a letter is unaware of the marital status of a female recipient, he shall not address her as 'Dear Ms.' He shall instead start the letter 'Dear Madam.' " Grant blew his breath through his lips with distended cheeks like Jack Frost making a winter wind. He held up the constitution. "You will notice that 'madam' is spelled without an 'e.' 'Madam' without an 'e' means the keeper of a brothel. In effect, the recipient of such a letter, possibly an innocent young girl, is being accused of running a whorehouse."

"Make the motion," said Akt. He sounded near exhaustion.

"I move," said Grant, mopping his forehead with a clean handkerchief, "that on page thirty-six 'madam' be spelled with an 'e.' "

The motion was passed with speed and indifference.

"I think that this is important," said Grant doggedly.

"I do too," said Akt, "so important, in fact, that we should continue these revisions when we can devote more time to them."

"Caries," said Scotti, "you should have been at the Constitutional Convention in Philadelphia two hundred years ago. Then we wouldn't have to listen to you now."

Akt tapped on the table with his pen. "Let's get on with the meeting. Last time I appointed a search committee consisting of Doctors Bligh, Grant, and Scotti, with Bligh as chairman. May we have the report, please?"

Bligh picked up a pencil as if it were a scalpel but his tremor forced him to replace it on the table. "There were thirty-two applicants, all of unusually high caliber. They came from as far away as Philadelphia. Evidently the medical profession finds a position on this board far from unattractive. The committee personally interviewed twenty-three of these pediatricians. After a careful screening and many prolonged discussions, we were able to unanimously recommend two candidates, in alphabetical order, Dr. Keats and Dr. Wells."

"We all realize how much work this must have entailed," said Akt. "Thank you."

He nodded to Bligh, who moved that the report be adopted. The seven directors mumbled their approval.

"Before we vote on the two candidates," said Akt, "I am going to open the floor for discussion."

There was an awkward silence. Even though nothing that would be said would change anyone's vote, short, sponsoring speeches were considered necessary. This was the tribute which the closed mind paid to tradition.

Bligh raised his right hand not so much to obtain permission to speak as to make sure that his colleagues listened attentively. It shook a little.

"We must decide this afternoon whether we will cling to the past or embrace the future; whether we will advance with Wells or retreat with Keats. Wells was trained in the Medical Center. He is one of Professor Locke's bright young men. He has rejuvenated the Department of Pediatrics by increasing the resident staff to fourteen and mapping out a program for their education which is a marvel of ingenuity. His practice is enormous; Keats's, by comparison, is minute. There must be a reason for the community's preference. All these patients can't be wrong. True, Wells is much younger than any of us, but that makes him all the more remarkable. We are interested in the future of Adams. This man offers great promise for the days to come."

"I'm not impressed by the I.O.U. of promise," said Ray. "I prefer the hard cash of accomplishment."

Scotti raised his hand and said with a sardonic smile, "I wouldn't say that Wells is lacking in accomplishments. He's increased the number of residents to fourteen when six could do the job much better. That's an accomplishment. He's screwed more married women than any other man at Adams. That's an accomplishment. He's spent more money on income-tax-deductible entertainment than anyone here. That's an accomplishment. He's managed to avoid writing a single article or making one contribution to the scientific literature. That's an accomplishment."

Scotti took a deep breath and looked around the room. "Of course, Jim Keats has some accomplishments to his credit, too, but they are of a different kind. He's the best clinician the department has. He's written twenty-four articles, some of which were and still are of considerable significance. He introduced exchange transfusions to this hospital and later trained young men to perform them expertly. He is a master of the medical literature. And he has served Adams for thirty years. Of course, he's not pretty, like Wells." Here Scotti twisted his broken nose. "But then we old football players don't go in for looks."

He flashed his wolfish grin at his colleagues. "There is one more thing I would like to mention. Dr. Wells was Corky Guthrie's pediatrician. I use the past tense advisedly. The Mayo Clinic and the Children's Medical Center in Boston made the diagnosis of Dawson's encephalitis, a uniformly fatal disease. When Wells got the reports, he told the Guthries that he would cure their son with a solution of interferon more powerful than any yet developed." He put his hands and elbows on the table and looked around the room. "Do you know what the interferon solution really was? I have it on excellent authority that it was just ordinary, normal, saline solution. You don't believe me? Ask anyone what effect it had on the boy. None. Then Jim Keats injected a virus killer with which he has had considerable experience. The result was miraculous. The boy was cured." He looked around him again. "Can you see Wells running a million-dollar department of virology? All he would turn out would be a lot of saline solution fizzed up with his own hot air."

No one said anything for almost a minute. Then Akt asked, "Is there any further discussion?"

"Keats is fifty-four and a senior man," said Bligh. "We would have to pay him thirty-five thousand dollars a year. Wells is young and has an independent income. We could probably get him for twenty-five."

Scotti turned toward the president of the medical board. "You would think Bligh was going to pay the salary of the new director of Pediatrics out of his own pocket."

Akt tapped on the table with his ballpoint pen. It was a Cross and was beginning to show a dent on top. "Let's get on with the meeting. Dummer?" he asked.

"I am convinced that Wells would do an excellent job," said the Director of Pediatrics. "He has for me."

"Grant?"

"Wells gets along with people," said the Director of Laboratories. "That's what counts."

"Airov?"

The Director of Anesthesia responded with a guileless smile. "No comment."

Akt nodded to Grant. "Then we will vote."

The secretary of the medical board passed around three-inch squares of blank white paper on which each director wrote the name of his choice. Each then folded the paper carefully and slid it back across the table to Grant. The secrecy of the ballot was respected even though it would become obvious how every member had voted the moment the tabulations were completed. Grant unfolded and smoothed out the pieces of paper and made little marks in a note-book without changing his expression. Then, leaving the ballots on the table where they could be inspected by anyone who doubted his honesty, he announced,

"Four votes for Wells, three for Keats."

There was a long silence while each side considered its Pyrrhic victory.

"I can't speak for the trustees," said Hexter at last. "I'm just an employee like the elevator operators, the cooks, the porters, and you. But I am certain that the board will not accept this recommendation. The vote is too close."

"I see bad times ahead," said Akt. "This is the foot in the door. The trustees will increasingly take over the functions that belong to the doctors. They will be giving orders about purely medical matters. Don't you agree, Frank?"

"I'm afraid you're right," said Ray, trying to suppress a cough. "Only this time in addition to the usual jockeying for power a philo-sophical question has been raised. What kind of a man should be made the chief of a department? Your concept, Courtney, is that a young man should be brought in from another hospital, a young man with different ideas and fresh methods. My ideas are much more old-fashioned. I feel that the job should go to that member of the senior attending staff who most deserves it, to the department's outstanding physician. I think it is immoral for a hospital to encourage a doctor to work for it for thirty years only to snatch away the prize in the end and present it to a young stranger."

"Putting philosophy and morality aside for a moment," said Hexter, "I think you ought to consider the trustees' point of view on such a close vote for a director. The first story I heard about this medical board illustrates my point rather well. My informant tells me that an extremely unpopular attending—we don't have to mention his name —had a prostatectomy several years ago. He says you sent the patient a note which read: 'At its last meeting the medical board passed a resolution wishing you a speedy recovery. The vote was four to three.' Now, gentlemen, in certain situations a four-to-three vote is not good enough. The trustees will not accept it for a position as important as the directorship of a major department. I don't mean to be offensive, but they are getting tired of your constant bickering. Can't you unite behind a single candidate?"

Akt looked at Airov and said, "Does anybody want to change his mind?"

The anesthetist turned on his broad, peasant smile and said, "No, nobody wants to change his mind."

The following morning Joseph Crunch, the chairman of the board of trustees, telephoned Dr. Akt that there would be a special meeting of the joint conference committee on Monday, the thirty-first of December, at three o'clock. The seven trustees had decided, he said, to interview both Dr. Keats and Dr. Wells themselves. The president of the medical board resolved to show some independence.

"New Year's Eve, you say? That's only four days away. I don't know whether the other directors and I can come on such short notice."

Crunch laughed. "This time you can't tell me you're operating. The nursing supervisor says you're not on the schedule. Neither is Bligh. But if you can't come, you can't come. You're a busy man and we'll have to get along without you. But try. For thirty-five thousand dollars a year I think you should try."

Akt promised that he would.

Crunch had a poor opinion of most of the Adams doctors, especially the younger ones. In Mr. Gulbanian's day the attendings had devoted half of their time to treating the poor of the City of New

York on the wards and in the clinics free of charge. But Medicare and Medicaid had changed all that. Today, in his opinion, the doctors were adequately paid for taking care of the old and the indigent. And the directors, all of whom had large private practices, received thirty-five grand a year for doing what their predecessors had been eager to do for nothing.

He thought even less of the trustees. In Mr. Gulbanian's day a trustee was a philanthropist. Tom Guthrie and a half dozen others measured up to this definition. The rest were nickel-nursers, he said to himself. The thirty-man board included a minister, a sociologist, a leader of the community—whatever the hell that was, an economist, an appointed government official, the son of a former governor of Maine, a lawyer, a few members of socially prominent families, a half dozen retired officers of corporations, and a black professor of romance languages. He was a lovely man and had been elected to show that Adams was a liberal institution. You couldn't find a loose dollar in a carload of people like that, Crunch said to himself in disgust.

Five years earlier he had been asked by the board of trustees to come to Adams and save it from bankruptcy. On going over the books he had been appalled to discover that the doctors, who according to custom had never before been asked to open their checkbooks since after all there were certainly no great financiers among them, this time had been dragooned into raising one million dollars toward the construction of a new building. The trustees, on the other hand, the so-called philanthropists who in return for the honored title were supposed to support their hospital, couldn't be persuaded to part with more than half a million. Nevertheless, he took the job. He felt that he owed Adams something. Twenty-eight years before, when he was nineteen, his mother had been admitted to the free surgical wards with cancer of the breast. Three months later his father had followed her with an acutely inflamed gall bladder. The young man had never forgotten the devotion, the skill, the warmth, and the kindness with which the physicians, surgeons, interns, and nurses had treated his parents in those prewar days. He felt he had to do something to pay them back.

The first thing he did was to bring in half a dozen men who would have passed muster before Mr. Gulbanian. They became the givers. The rest of the trustees made speeches, gave advice, showed up at the meetings, voted the way they were told, and bought tickets for the benefits. He did not think much of them. He also did not think much of diplomacy either; wheeling and dealing, negotiating and debating, yes, but not diplomacy, which he equated with tweedy gentlemen, weakness or Borgia poisons. In four years he had raised Adams to its feet. The nongiving trustees put up with his coarseness and insults because they knew that without him the hospital would have perished. They excused him and pretended that they were not offended, saying that he was a rough diamond with a heart of gold, a remark which prompted him to reply that they were confusing him with Tiffany's.

Joe Crunch had been born and raised in the Bronx. He had supported himself while attending City College, a tuition-free institution, by collecting garbage on the dawn shift for a private disposal company. The Plaza was the most important customer on his route. As he lugged the heavy cans from the hotel to the truck he vowed that someday he would contribute to that garbage instead of carrying it. He kept his word. Once a year he and his wife would leave their Fifth Avenue duplex apartment to spend a weekend at the Plaza. The moment they crossed the threshold of their suite he would bellow, "Molly, we're going to contribute to some of the finest garbage in the City of New York. Only this time I won't have to cart it away." Then they would throw everything they could think of into the trash baskets and eat large meals in the hotel's dining rooms, concentrating on foods which left a large residue, like melons, bananas, lobster, and duck.

He had made his money in construction and real estate. By 1973 he was worth forty million dollars. His once-black, wiry hair now looked like a dusty brush. But he was still muscular and unwrinkled. His head was still fixed in an almost constant upward tilt because he felt that the next person he met would tower above him. And it was still cocked a little to one side, the better to estimate his adversaries. He regarded most men and a few women as potential adversaries. And he still smoked thick black cigars although he knew that a pipe or even cigarettes would make him look more like a gentleman. Recently during conferences he had acquired the infuriating habit of dropping his ashes into the ashtrays of those sitting on either side of him, leaving his own ashtray spotless. This was probably the result of his youthful experiences. Let the others gaze at the garbage, he seemed to be saying. I saw enough of it in the old days. Briefed by Tom Guthrie, he looked forward with pleasure to the two interviews on the thirty-first.

The morning after Crunch had telephoned the president of the board, Jim sat in Trudy's office. It was exactly quarter to eight and she had been waiting for him.

"The game is going into sudden-death overtime," he said. "The joint conference committee is interviewing Wells and me next Monday afternoon. I'm sure that's when the trustees will make up their minds. To add to the excitement they have decided to set up a department of virology as soon as they can raise another half million. You won't believe it, but it's going to be under the control of the new director of Pediatrics. This directorship is going to be a very important position."

"Jimmy, when you get your divorce, don't you want to get married again, this time for good? Don't you want some woman to love you?"

"If she only would."

"She will, but you will have to protect her, take care of her, support her. You will have to insist that she never works again even though she insists that she wants to. That means you have got to get this job. Please don't go passive and do yourself in with medical ethics when the trustees grill you on Monday. You're too big to be a mouse. And please don't be loyal to your chief, that insufferable ass, E-e-evan Dummer. He's the one who brought Wells here in the first place. And please don't forget who tried to steal your virus killer. I just hope you brand him with the scarlet letter, not the A for adultery but the T for thief."

For a moment he thought of Annie Laurie, of the slim, almost emaciated model's body, of the skin drawn tight over the aristocratic facial bones which had been created and molded in a slum in Queens, of the sleek black hair and the cold black eyes which never once lit up when they rested on him. Cold and tight and ready to fight, that was his Annie Laurie. He gazed at the big beautiful blonde woman on the other side of the desk, twelve years older than his wife but an ageless fifty, at the violet eyes and creamy skin, at the white expanse of uniform which concealed what once must have been a ravishing body, and felt the warmth and womanliness radiating from her that no mantle of efficiency could conceal. He stood up and placed the tips of his fingers on the desk.

"Trudy, I'm going to hit the line Monday afternoon. I haven't forgotten how."

The door was open but no one was passing by. He leaned over and kissed her on the lips.

16

By FOUR P.M. Monday the thirty-first of December 1973, fifteen men were seated around the table in the big council room at Adams. There were the seven directors. Crunch had been right. Reminded of their thirty-five-thousand-dollar-a-year salaries, they had all been quick to discover that there were no conflicting appointments in their calendars. There was Hexter, the administrator, who was attempting to make "compassion" a four-letter word at Adams. An article about his regime could well have been entitled "The Death of the Heart." It was he who had instituted the system in which the patients were forced to write out their checks for estimated expenses one week in advance, thereby conforming to his philosophy which was pay now, die later. And what if they should live? So much the better. They could come back and pay one week in advance again. And finally there were the only ones who really counted at this meeting, the seven trustees, Crunch, four of the six philanthropically minded men he had brought with him, his friend, Tom Guthrie, and Neville Narr, one of the noncontributors whom the chairman had placed at his right so that he could drop ashes into his ashtray. Once during a meeting of the board of directors of a steel corporation Crunch had attempted to play this trick on Wright, the Medical Center's illustrious philanthropist who was reputed to be worth almost a billion dollars. The old man had waited until a heated argument had broken out. Then he had deftly exchanged ashtrays. Crunch, who had felt that he ought to apologize but had not known how, had said, "I just wanted to see how far I could go." The old man had responded with a frosty smile. "With me? Not an inch." No one at Adams had ever dared to switch ashtrays with Crunch.

Neville Narr had been put on the conference committee because he typified those trustees whom Crunch characterized as window dressing. At sixty-three Narr was almost as handsome as he had been thirty-five years before, when he had come from England to New York with letters of recommendation to Phyffe and Drumme, even then one of the most important advertising companies in the country. Mr. Phyffe had hired him at once not merely because of his Churchillian English and suave bearing but because he had seen in him a husband for his thirty-year-old homely and vixenish daughter, who had so far proved unmarriageable. From the very first his co-workers had seen in him the silly ass, that vaudeville misrepresentation of an Englishman that was then fashionable among the lower classes. He became the butt of mild practical jokes. When during that first year he had asked the men in the office where he could buy a bowler, they had patiently explained to him that in New York men wore straw hats in June. Since he was not to be dissuaded, they recommended Knox, then on Fifth Avenue and Fortieth Street. He returned at the end of the lunch hour with a derby which had his initials stamped in gold in the hatband. The next morning one of the men at the office bought a hat at Knox similar in every respect down to the position of the initials except for the fact that it was three sizes larger. The two bowlers were quickly switched. When Narr put on his hat before going out to lunch, it came down over his ears. A careful examination revealed no cause for the catastrophe, one, fortunately, that he was able to surmount by lining the hatband with paper. The next morning his fellow workers brought out the derby he had originally purchased and transferred the paper to it. This time he could not get the hat down on his head. His composure was not strengthened when late that afternoon he overheard one of the copywriters tell a group that his brother had just left for Sweden to consult the world's greatest authority, in fact the only authority, on a strange disease characterized by alternate expansion and contraction of the skull.

Although Mr. Phyffe was aware of the general attitude toward Narr, one that mingled scorn with good-natured acceptance, he was satisfied with his employee's all-around performance since it was obviously excellent in the only area that counted. The young man had taken out the ugly duck (she was a duckling no longer) six times, three of them to a hotel, and they had gotten along well together. The following year they were married. The new Mrs. Narr's disposition immediately showed a vast improvement. Shortly after this Mr. Phyffe discovered that two of his junior executives had devised an elaborate scheme for siphoning off some of the company's money into their own pockets. He called them before him and told them that he had to let them go. He did not say why. They knew. Very courteously he asked whether they had any plans for the immediate future. Yes, they replied, they were going into business for themselves. And the name of their new firm? he inquired. As yet they had none. He coughed discreetly.

"I can suggest one that is both dignified and catchy. Why not call it 'Fagin and Sykes'?" When they seemed puzzled, he added, "From *Oliver Twist,* the two biggest crooks in Dickens' novels."

He awarded one of the two positions vacated by the pair to Narr; the other to an old employee.

"Your job," he said to the latter, "will be to teach my son-in-law how to put one foot in front of the other. And don't let him fall on his penis. It's my daughter's pride and joy."

After this Neville's rise had been rapid although his duties remained vague. When the old man died in 1965, he was made chairman of the board with no responsibilities and no power. Phyffe's two sons ran the business. Narr decided that his primary duty was to keep up the traditions of the firm. One of them was the tour of the sixty-three offices which for thirty years Mr. Phyffe had made on the day before Christmas. He would visit them and not only wish the occupants a merry Christmas but greet every one of them by name, a feat he was able to accomplish not because of a superb memory but because of the nameplates which were screwed into all the doors. When Narr became chairman of the board, frequent hirings and firings as well as changes in assignments had resulted in slots replacing the screws. Each year a few minutes before he made his pre-Christmas grand tour, the men would remove the nameplates and substitute others from different offices. He would then start his rounds, purr, "Merry Christmas," and call every employee by someone else's name. Then everybody would go to the party and get drunk.

Both Crunch and Guthrie considered Neville one of the most important men at Adams, not because of brains or generosity but because of the very lack of them. He was a composite of two thirds of the board, they felt, revealing his colleagues' impotence in faithful detail. The philanthropist trustee of the first half of the twentieth century had been replaced by the microgiver of the second. Munificence was in short supply. Big spenders were hard to find. Yet the hospital had to fill its roster of trustees. To fail to do so would have put it in the position of a charitable organization which sent out an appeal for funds with the names of only two or three sponsors on its letterhead. Adams elected to its board second-rate sons of first-rate fathers, political appointees, old-timers who were over the hill and about to retire from positions in banking and industry, and anyone with a name which might bring prestige to the hospital. Their monetary contributions were token. Neville Narr had impeccable credentials—social standing, membership in good clubs, a terribly important-sounding position in a powerful advertising agency, a flawless voting record since he always did as he was told, and an empty wallet as far as Adams was concerned. Besides, he always bought two tickets for the benefits. He was the perfect embodiment of the new trustee, a worthy representative of the other twenty. That was why he had been appointed to the joint conference committee.

Crunch sat at the head of the table in the big council room with Narr on his right, their ashtrays immaculate. The other five trustees, in well-cut business suits, were grouped nearby. The seven doctors in starched white coats had taken their places at the other end of the table, leaving a significant gap, however, between themselves and Hexter, who sat at the foot. It was as if they wished to avoid his chilling personality on this icy December day. But there was another reason for their aloofness. As far back as anyone could remember, Adams had always taken care of its old doctors when they were sick. Blue Cross and more recently Medicare paid for a semiprivate room. But the old attendings, like everyone else, yearned for blessed privacy so that they would not have to share the noises of defecation, urination, and flatus with a strange roommate. The hospital had never failed to put them in private rooms at no extra cost to repay them for all the free work they had done in years gone by. Recently Hexter had decided that there would be no discounts for Adams doctors. Many of the old attendings were still practicing in a gallant attempt to make ends meet. Many suffered cruel financial losses when a hospital stay prevented them from earning a living. The directors did not pull their chairs away from Hexter or pointedly disassociate themselves from him. On the other hand, they did not feel he was the kind of man they wanted to sit too close to.

Joe Crunch lit a fat black cigar, tilted his head a little further to the side, the better to take the measure of the directors, and said,

"I see that in spite of busy schedules all the men in white have managed to come to the meeting, even those who are a little gray around the edges. Up here we also have one hundred percent attendance. That is important because we represent the other trustees." He leaned forward as if to impart a confidence and whispered hoarsely, "One of them just gave up his American Express card so that he could donate the fifteen dollars a year to Adams."

He reached over and dropped ashes in Neville Narr's ashtray. Then he turned to Courtney Akt and said, "Get Dr. Keats in, please."

Akt reached for the telephone.

A moment later Jim walked in looking tough and enormous as he passed through the doorway. He had taken off ten pounds from his middle and was down to two hundred and thirty. Joe Crunch liked men this big because they made not only him but everyone else look small.

"Doctor," he said after Jim sat down and put an attaché case on the table, "I used to see you carry the ball for Columbia when I was a kid. You haven't changed. I'll bet you could still play."

Jim gave him a crooked smile. "Sure, sure, I haven't changed, but those linesmen have suddenly become big, mean, and young."

"Would you play if number Seventy-three opened up those holes for you again?"

Jim looked at Scotti. "Maybe then."

"Dr. Keats," said Crunch, "I've read your record on and off the field and heard about you from Mr. Guthrie. But we have never met. This afternoon I would like to get to know you a little better."

Neville Narr laughed. "It's like that song from *The King and I,* 'Getting to Know You.' Not bad, eh?"

Crunch reached out and dumped ashes in Narr's ashtray. "Bad," he said severely. He turned to Jim. "We would like to hear some of your opinions, on, well, almost anything." He paused. "What do you think of the future of Adams? Are you optimistic or pessimistic?"

"Pessimistic," answered Jim. "I think we are approaching the end of the golden age of medicine. It's hard to realize but doctors have accomplished more in the past fifty years than in all the centuries since the beginning of time. I hope that the next fifty years will be as productive. I am afraid, though, that they will mark the end of what makes medicine an art as well as a science—the good doctor-patient relationship. Medicine as we know it today will be destroyed, not by any deficiencies of the doctors or by excessive demands by the patients but by that money-devouring monster, the hospital. Growing constantly more voracious as it eats up bigger and bigger chunks of the financial resources of the sick, it will end up by pulling the entire structure of medicine down on all of us, doctors, patients, and trustees alike. People simply cannot afford to pay two hundred dollars a day for a private room or one hundred dollars a day for a bed on the so-called free wards. The middle class will no longer accept a bill of ten thousand dollars for a six-weeks' stay that does not include adequate nursing care. Sure, Blue Cross and Major Medical will pay most of it, but they have to charge premiums which are rising out of sight. The hospitals are pricing themselves out of the market. Eventually they will be taken over by the institution that has the greatest unbroken experience with waste and extravagance."

"And what is that?" asked Narr naively.

"The government. Hospital care will be paid for by taxation, which the people always accept as they do their own mortality."

"Dr. Keats," said Tom Guthrie, "you mentioned waste and extravagance. Do you think there is much of that here?"

"Yes, but a lot of it is unavoidable. It is extravagant for a charitable institution to pay a man one hundred and sixty dollars a week for a simple, menial job, but it is a necessary extravagance. You can't expect him to work for twenty-five dollars a week the way his father once did. But if he gives the hospital eighty dollars' worth of work a week for the one hundred and sixty, that is an unnecessary extravagance and the administrator should do something about it."

Crunch tilted his neck to the side, looked hard at Hexter sitting stiffly at the other end of the table, and said, "He certainly should. And apropos of what you just said, Doctor, the elevator service here stinks."

Jim waited respectfully for a moment and continued, "A good hospital must train and pay a lot of residents. It's a modern custom.

The four years they spend here must be recognized as an extension of medical school. Only nobody ever flunks out since no exams are ever given. Eighteen-thousand-dollar-a-year residents are a necessary extravagance. But if you have twice as many as you need, that's an unnecessary extravagance. Adams could get along with half as many residents as it now has and save almost a million dollars a year in the bargain." He gave Hexter a mean look. "That's enough to give private rooms to our sick old doctors so that they can recover in luxury or die in peace. And there would still be a lot of money left over."

Neville Narr harumphed. "But, Doctor, don't you think we have to train these young men? After all, we have a duty to the community."

"Do you think that after we finish with these young men they will practice in the community? Or in Watts, Harlem, Appalachia, and the other poverty-stricken sections of our country which need them so desperately?" He snorted. "They set up their shingles in the affluent suburbs. Or else they return to the underprivileged countries which are constantly reviling us or to the Middle Eastern kingdoms which blackmail us with their oil. Did you ever hear of one of those billionaire petroleum potentates making a contribution to Adams to show his gratitude?"

"No, come to think of it, I never did," admitted Narr.

An ambulance siren sounded close by, announcing, perhaps, said Jim to himself, that an unconscious victim of an automobile accident, or a middle-aged man with the unbearable pain of a coronary occlusion, or a woman sledge-hammered by a stroke was being brought to Adams. He thought of the patients who were about to undergo cesarean sections, operations for the removal of the stomach, prostate, or much of the large intestine, of the neurosurgeons who would unsuccessfully attempt to extirpate brain tumors, and of the poor souls with terminal cancer who would uncomplainingly take chemotherapy every day. And a rage came over him at the realization that waste, sloppiness, and extravagance were depriving the sick of money necessary for their care and for the research which might someday lead to discoveries which could have cured them.

He turned to the chairman of the board, who looked to him like a benign courtroom judge, and said calmly,

"One of the most flagrant examples of extravagance, Mr. Crunch, is the overutilization of the diagnostic machines. We have one called the SMA 12, which costs seventy-five thousand dollars and does twelve blood chemistries simultaneously on every patient whether he needs them or not, a luxury we rationalize by saying that as long as we are doing one we might as well do twelve. This is a necessary extravagance. It is called automation. Every hospital in the country has such a machine and uses it on patients whether they have dandruff or appendicitis. What is an unnecessary extravagance is checklist medicine, so loved by the house staff, in which the doctor orders every X-ray and laboratory test the hospital is equipped to perform under the theory that in this way he will be less likely to miss any clue that might lead to a diagnosis. In the old days the master clinician would stop at the bed of a drowsy patient, smell acetone on his breath, and confirm the diagnosis of diabetes by ordering a blood sugar and a CO_2. Those days will never return. I shudder to think of a future in which an SMA 500 will turn out five hundred tests simultaneously, four hundred ninety-nine of which are unnecessary, and feed them into a computer. As the machines grow larger, the doctors' brains will grow smaller until they will finally wither away with the atrophy of disuse. Of course, there is nothing wrong with the machines any more than there is anything wrong with a Steinway piano, an atomic reactor, or a high-spirited horse. It's the men who misuse them who should be censured. Unfortunately, no one will ever build a machine which will be able to comfort the mother of a dying child."

"Thank you, Doctor," said Crunch. "We understand." He dropped some ashes in Neville Narr's ashtray. "What do you think of the way the Department of Pediatrics is now being run?"

Jim opened his attaché case and held up a sheaf of Xeroxed pages. "It's a paper service. These pages are filled with the names of doctors. When a young man finishes his residency here, he is automatically given a position on the attending staff as long as he practices within fifty miles of the hospital. He doesn't have to earn the appointment. It just helps make the service look big and important. Some of these doctors haven't been seen here in a year." He looked through the pages. "Take this, for instance. A different junior attending is on call every night of the week. He is supposed to respond to emergencies. Can you imagine any of these fellows driving over icy roads from Westchester or Long Island at two in the morning to see a free ward case? They haven't been to Adams in so long they couldn't find the way. Nevertheless, they are listed here as being on active duty. They are as active as a bunch of toy soldiers. You have to admit, though, that the schedule looks impressive.

"Worse than this, though, has been the destruction of the backbone of the service, the experienced attendings between forty and sixty. They have been banished from the department. Not so long ago they made rounds regularly three to four times a week. Now they are on the schedule only once a month."

"Who is responsible for this paper facade?" asked Guthrie.

Jim did not answer at once. "I'm a team man and I don't like to mention names. Let's just say it's been erected by the new regime."

"Every new regime has a founder," Guthrie pressed on relentlessly. "Who started this one?"

Jim hesitated. "You might say Dr. Wells."

Neville Narr harumphed. "I thought Dr. Dummer was the director."

"He is," answered Jim, "but his junior partner is the gray eminence."

"How was a young man like Dr. Wells able to acquire such power?" asked Guthrie.

"He is the paper man, and on the Department of Pediatrics the pen is mightier than the ward. He draws up these impressive schedules which make the service look good and push us older men aside at the same time. I have served Adams for thirty years and I haven't been allowed to make rounds in a month. The Department of Pediatrics has become a two-class society consisting of the director and his gray eminence on the one hand and the residents on the other. Rounds are made almost exclusively by Dr. Dummer and the fourteen drones. The others, and that includes all the experienced attendings, are supposed to stay away."

"That's a good way to get rid of the competition," said Crunch, puffing on his cigar, "but it seems to me like a helluva way to run a service."

Guthrie pawed through some papers. Then he raised his head. He reminded Jim of a bloodhound getting a scent. "Dr. Keats, would you mind telling us what goes on behind the paper facade?"

Jim looked around him slowly. "Well, the weekly conferences are poorly attended. Research is never mentioned much less attempted. There is little teaching by the experienced members of the staff. The nurseries are cute, but no investigative work ever comes out of them. The seminars are unable to produce a much-to-be-desired daytime insomnia among the house staff. The beds are in large measure empty. No one dies of overwork."

He raised the pages he was holding. "But you would never guess it from looking at the paper facade. If you took the trouble to read through these announcements with their duty rosters, nights on and nights off, weekends on and weekends off, seminars, speakers, ward rounds, nursery rounds, resident rounds, sign-out rounds (at four P.M., if you please), schedules, conferences, and outpatient clinics, you would be convinced that our Department of Pediatrics was greater than the Harvard Children's Medical Center. Actually, I'm sorry to say, it's hardly worth the paper it's written on."

Dummer cleared his throat. "I'd like to say something in defense of the department."

"It's Dr. Keats we are interviewing this afternoon," said Crunch, tapping more ashes into Narr's ashtray. His own was spotless. "It seems as if the Department of Pediatrics could use the services of a good garbage man. I used to be one, so I know."

"Dr. Keats," said Tom Guthrie, "everyone in the hospital seems to be talking about your virus killer, I perhaps more than most because it saved my son's life. Could you tell us about it?"

"It's a long story," said Jim. "I don't know whether you have the time."

"We've listened to so much crap in this room," said Crunch, "it will be a pleasure to hear something important for a change."

Jim nodded and patiently began to recount the story of the virus killer, how the mad technician had created a concoction an addled brain could never duplicate, how Professor Choate had given it to his old classmate under the impression that it was pure interferon, how he had tried it on a dog with distemper and then on himself, how it had saved the lives of three children who without it would have died, and how the Medical Center with all its resources had been unable to discover its formula.

The trustees and doctors were stunned.

"How much do you have left?" asked Crunch.

"One dose," Jim answered.

"Do you mean to tell me," said Neville Narr, "that a mad technician came up with a drug that has eluded the best brains in medicine?"

Jim shrugged. "Perhaps there is a touch of madness in every genius."

Narr thought back to his youth. It had been sheer madness, he knew, for him, then a penniless English lad, to have suggested to the boss's daughter that she go out with him. Yet she had. It had been sheer madness for him to have asked her to marry him. Yet she had accepted his proposal. The marriage had turned out to be a good one, with plenty of sexual intercourse, three children, and no cheating. And it had undoubtedly helped him in his career. He brushed some lint from the cuff of his jacket and looked up.

"Yes, perhaps there is a touch of madness in every genius," he said with pride. He hesitated for a moment. "I wish we had a product like yours at the agency instead of those bloody facial creams and gas-guzzling automobiles."

Crunch stubbed out his cigar in Narr's ashtray.

"Great discoveries are sometimes made by accident," Jim continued. "In 1928 in a London lab a mold fell purely by chance or perhaps through carelessness on a culture of microorganisms growing on a petri dish. When Alexander Fleming—the 'Sir' came later—examined the contaminated culture, he noticed that something emanating from the mold was destroying the germs. The mold was *Penicillium notatum*. The 'something' was penicillin. Fleming, Fleury, and Chaim put in a lot of work before they were able to isolate, purify, and mass produce it. But they did. The virus killer, too, was picked up by chance. Someday scientists will isolate, purify, and mass produce it. In the meantime all we can do is serenade it with Mr. Narr's favorite song, 'Getting to Know You,' and work like hell."

"Not bad," said Neville Narr.

Crunch smiled. "This time I agree with you—not bad."

"It's more than that," said Guthrie. "It's fascinating."

"So was the attempt to steal it," said Jim.

"Did you say 'steal it,' old man?" asked Narr in amazement. "Didn't you have it well secured?"

"Oh, yes, it was in a padlocked refrigerator in my laboratory in a bottle labeled 'Interferon.' That was what Professor Choate thought it was when he gave it to me."

"Who do you think tried to steal it?" asked Guthrie. When Jim did not answer at once, he continued, "Was it someone from Adams?"

"Yes, it was," answered Jim.

"Can't you be more specific?" demanded Guthrie. "Can't you give us a name?"

Jim hesitated. "It was Dr. Wells."

"That's a grave charge," said Guthrie after a moment. "Why would he take such a risk?"

"First, for the money. You will recall how generous you were in Corky's case. Second, to further his career. He's much better about publicity than I am. And third, to make sure that he would be the next director of Pediatrics. Besides, he had cooked up such a clever scheme that he figured there was virtually no risk."

"I see," said Guthrie. "But do you have any proof that Dr. Wells was involved?"

Jim reached into his attaché case and pulled out a piece of cloth. "A short time ago I went to a pediatric convention in Boston. I believe that one night while I was away Dr. Wells sneaked into my laboratory and stepped on the dog in the dark. That's certainly a reasonable supposition because when I returned I found the animal lying on his pad next to my desk with this between his paws. It is from my colleague's most flamboyant suit, and, as you can see, is of excellent quality."

He handed the specimen to Guthrie, who examined it thoroughly and passed it to the trustees.

"But, Doctor, this merely indicates that Dr. Wells entered your laboratory one night," said Guthrie. "It doesn't prove that he got into the refrigerator where the virus killer was stored. Your point is that he did break into the refrigerator, is it not?"

Jim nodded.

"Was the padlock sawed through?" asked Guthrie.

"No, it wasn't."

"Then someone besides you must have had a key," the trustee said. "I'm afraid you will have to tell us who it was."

"My wife," said Jim.

There was a long, intense silence.

For the first time Guthrie seemed taken aback. "Do you mean to say that Dr. Wells stole the key from your wife, and then used it to open your refrigerator one night while you were away?"

"No, I'm sure she opened the refrigerator for him."

Neville Narr harumphed and raised his handsome old head. "I'm from England, you know, and perhaps I am not as smart as you Yanks, but I don't see why she would want to do that."

"Let me explain it to you, Mr. Narr, as delicately as I can," said Scotti from the other end of the table. "Wells is a notorious charmer of married women."

Narr turned toward Jim. He seemed astounded. "Then you think that your wife and this other fellow may have been intimate."

"Neville!" warned Crunch, and there was an edge in his voice. "We are not going to pursue that line of questioning at this meeting."

He lit another fat black cigar, only, Jim was convinced, so that he could drop more ashes in Narr's ashtray.

"Oh, dear," said Narr, looking guilty. "I didn't mean to pry into anyone's family life."

"Dr. Keats," said Guthrie, "I would like to go a step further in unearthing the facts. You have stated that Dr. Wells entered your laboratory one night while you were away and opened the refrigerator with a key. I don't think it is necessary to ascertain how he got the key. I would like to know, however, what he found when he opened the refrigerator. Empty shelves?"

"Oh, no. He found a bottle labeled 'Interferon,'" said Jim. "The clever scheme he now put into effect made the entire operation practically foolproof. He poured the contents of my bottle into one he had brought with him. Then he replaced the fluid he had stolen from my bottle with an equal quantity of ordinary saline solution. Saline solution and the virus killer look exactly alike. There was no way I could have detected the theft on my return. Finally, he locked the refrigerator and walked out with the contents of my bottle and, unfortunately for him, a rip in his trousers."

"A very clever idea," said Narr, "one that required great imagination. That fellow would have gone far in the advertising world."

"You don't seem perturbed at the loss of your virus killer, Dr. Keats," said Crunch, cocking his head to one side. "You must have had an even slicker scheme up your sleeve."

Jim smiled. "I couldn't let him get away with it. Just before I went to Boston, it was suggested to me that Dr. Wells might attempt to steal the virus killer while I was away. Naturally, I took it out of my laboratory refrigerator and put it in a safe place. To give Wells a taste of his own medicine, I substituted a bottle identical in every respect into which I had poured some harmless saline solution. When my colleague raided my laboratory that night, he transferred my salt solution into a container of his own, thinking that he had gotten hold of the virus killer. Then he poured some salt solution into my empty bottle to cover the theft. Actually, all he was accomplishing was to replace one batch of saline solution with another."

Crunch laughed. "I've heard of fighting fire with fire, but never saline with saline. Beautiful, Doctor, beautiful."

Tom Guthrie looked grave. "But, Dr. Keats, do you have any proof of this?"

"Yes, I do," answered Jim. "Before I left, I wiped off the bottle in my refrigerator so that it would take fingerprints. When I returned, it was covered with Dr. Wells's fingerprints," he let out his breath, "and my wife's."

He reached into his attaché case and passed a Xeroxed copy of Captain Prince's report to each trustee. "The work was done by the head of the fingerprint division of the New York City Police Department. Miss Trudy Starr, the pediatric nursing supervisor, vouched for the authenticity of the exhibits. I think some of you know Miss Starr."

"We all do," said Crunch. "I agree to take her word. It is as good as a government bond under Coolidge."

"The lady is even better than her word," said Narr. "To anyone who has ever seen her she is much more exciting than a government bond under Coolidge." He looked at the chairman of the board hopefully. "Not bad, eh?"

Crunch shook his head in despair. "Bad," he said.

The trustees read their copies of the report carefully.

When they were finished Jim said to Guthrie, "The reason why Dr. Wells couldn't help Corky was that he injected ordinary saline solution into his vein."

Guthrie smiled. "You're a good detective."

"I've had enough experience," said Jim. "A doctor has to be a detective in the world of disease."

There was a long pause. Crunch reached across the table and shook Jim's hand.

"You've built up an impressive case, Doctor. I am convinced. And thank you for telling us things we should have been told before." He smiled. "This is not the first time old Forty-one made his hundred yards. Wait outside for a few minutes, will you?"

Jeez, said Jim to himself, he remembers my number. He took his attaché case and walked out, his shoulders filling the doorway.

Crunch sat down and said to Akt, "Get Wells, please."

The president of the medical board picked up the telephone.

Wells opened the door and walked in. He was handsome, slim, and tanned by the daily use of a sunlamp. The trustees were too fascinated by his suit, however, to notice his physical characteristics. It had been an unfortunate choice since it was obviously the very one from which the piece of fabric they had just been handling had been torn.

As soon as he sat down Crunch turned toward him and said, "Doctor, what do you think of the future of Adams? Are you optimistic or pessimistic?"

"Optimistic," said Wells. "We have and always have had good doctors, administrators, and trustees. Most hospitals are situated in ghetto areas. That is as it should be. The poor must be taken care of. But the rich get sick, too. Fortunately, we are situated in one of the finest neighborhoods in New York. The community should be encouraged to make financial contributions toward our growth. I'm bullish on Adams. I just wish the stock market would follow our curve."

"Doctor, how do you think the Department of Pediatrics is being run?"

"Beautifully. I must confess that I have three fathers, my own, Dr. Locke of the Medical Center, and Dr. Dummer here. My Adams father has done a magnificent job. We have fourteen residents. No service of our size in the entire city has that many. And our educational program, seminars, conferences, rounds, and lectures keep them so busy that they don't have time to catch their breath. If I am fortunate enough to be made director, my motto will be, 'More of the same.' In addition, I think I can assure you that my connections with Professor Locke are so close that in a short time I will be able to effect an affiliation between my department and the medical school with clinical professorships for the members of our staff."

Dummer beamed.

"Doctor," said Crunch, "Dr. Keats has just accused you of stealing what you thought was a priceless, almost magical drug, a virus killer. Please listen carefully." With no omissions he repeated what Keats had told the joint conference committee a few minutes before. When he finished, he slid a Xeroxed copy of Captain Prince's report down the table. "Take as much time as you wish, Doctor."

The directors and the trustees doodled on the pads in front of them or consulted blank pages in memo books. After a little while Wells looked up and smiled.

"Do you have any comments?" asked Crunch.

"Yes," said Wells. "Everywhere I see the name of Miss Trudy Starr. She is the ubiquitous witness and verifier. Surely Dr. Keats must have some friends among the hundreds of men who work at Adams. Why didn't he choose one of them? I find it strange that a married man picked a woman to do his dirty work."

"Evil is in the eye of the beholder," said Guthrie.

Narr harumphed. "I hear that when it comes to the fair sex, you are a bit of a charmer yourself."

"A harmless exaggeration by envious rivals," retorted Wells. "Besides, I am not a married man."

A cool customer, thought Crunch. He cocked his head and asked, "Do you deny the accusation?"

"I ignore it," answered Wells. "I'm more concerned with determining whether I can bring a suit for slander."

"You can't win it if the accusations are true," said Guthrie.

"I think I will consult two of my patients who are considered to be among the most successful libel lawyers in the country."

There was a spasm of coughing near the foot of the table. Frank Ray removed a slightly bloodstained handkerchief from his lips. "You may need a lawyer before long."

"Perhaps," said Wells. "Still I cannot understand the attitude of the joint conference committee. From what has been said one would think that the thief, if indeed there was one, attempted to steal this virus killer in order to sell it to the highest bidder, unload it on a fence, or peddle it to a foreign power. I am sure that all he wanted to do was inject it into hopelessly ill children just as Dr. Keats did. But whereas my colleague conducted his operations in the strictest secrecy, as if there was something illicit about them, perhaps this other man would have given the virus killer the publicity it deserved for the greater glory of Adams."

"Doctor," said Crunch, "under the Constitution, not of Adams, which Dr. Grant is currently revising, but of the United States, the accused has the right to confront his accuser. Do you want me to re-call Dr. Keats so that you can answer his charges face to face?"

Wells raised his hand. "Please, no shouting matches, no wrangling. I don't want to descend to his level."

Crunch shrugged. "Since you don't want to descend, I guess all that remains is for you to ascend—from your chair, I mean. We won't keep you. We have no further questions. You, I suppose, have no further answers."

Wells rose, bowed, and walked out. To hell with them, he said to himself. Not a man on the service has a practice that can hold a can-dle to mine. So I was a fool to give Ann thirty-five thousand dollars. Maybe I'll find out that it is a legitimate tax deduction.

The trustees stared at his retreating figure as if they expected to find the place in his suit from which the piece of cloth they had just handled had been ripped.

Crunch addressed the doctors. "Would you be good enough to wait in the small conference room for a few minutes? And, Dr. Scotti, would you tell Dr. Keats we won't need him anymore today?"

The directors walked out slowly. As soon as they reached the cor-ridor Dummer took Airov by the arm and said,

"So you've won a famous victory! Good! Only you ruined the De-partment of Pediatrics in the process. Wells is Professor Locke's boy. A departmental affiliation with the medical school and the Medical Center would have followed his appointment as surely as the night the day."

Airov turned on his big muzhik smile. "Shakespeare?"

"Stop clowning, Leonid. I don't like to watch my department dis-integrate before my eyes."

"Stop weeping, Evan. Things are going to be much better this way."

"They are going to be much worse. Locke has been supplying us with our residents. That stream will dry up. We'll be a two-resident service in a couple of years."

"Evan, you're an argumentative, unconsolable, unregenerate pessimist. You should be quarantined."

Scotti and Jim walked past without greeting them. When they reached the end of the corridor Scotti said, "You cockalized the sonofabitch. I'll meet you in the doctors' lounge after the meeting."

Five minutes later the directors were summoned back to the council room. Crunch was still puffing on his thick black cigar.

"Gentlemen," he said as soon as they were seated, "we have decided not to consider Dr. Wells for the position. To put it bluntly, you have given us a bum steer, thrown us a curve ball. Dr. Scotti, exactly what did you mean when you said that Wells was a notorious charmer of married women?"

"I meant that he is a compulsive whoremaster who screws any married woman he can get up to his apartment," answered Scotti.

"Ah," said Crunch, "I see that five minutes with your colleagues has improved your vocabulary. I understand you perfectly now. In any case, Wells is through. I have appointed Mr. Guthrie as an ad hoc committee of one to canvass the medical schools and the hospitals of New York for additional suitable candidates. We were impressed with Dr. Keats. We think he is the man for the job." He dropped ashes into Narr's ashtray rather sadly, as if he realized that this was to be his last fling. "But we want to touch all the bases. Mr. Guthrie will report to the joint conference committee at the end of January. A happy 1974 to all of you."

Dummer, Bligh, Grant, and Akt looked as unhappy as men who have just laid a sizable bet on a losing horse. As a winner, Scotti felt he had the right to leave before anyone else. Jim was staring out the window in the doctors' lounge.

"The trustees think you are the man for the job," said Scotti, "but they are sending Tom Guthrie to look for talent in a few hospitals just for the record."

Jim frowned. "Do you think he will look very hard?"

Scotti laughed. "Are you kidding? You saved his son's life. You destroyed the opposition. What do you think?"

17

WHEN JIM came home at six that evening he saw a small suit-case resting against a chair in the foyer. Annie Laurie was standing at the other end of the living room.

"I'm spending the night with my sister and her family in Queens," she said. "It's not the Waldorf, but maybe we'll all have a few laughs."

She walked to the toilet. As soon as Jim heard the door click, he flipped open the valise. On top was an evening dress. Just what she needs for a family reunion in her sister's walk-up tenement, he said to himself. He closed the suitcase quickly and sat down to read the evening paper. She hurried through the living room to the foyer, picked up the valise, and closed the apartment door behind her with-out saying goodbye. Fifteen minutes later the doctor's answering service telephoned him to call Mr. Roach. The superintendent picked up the receiver on the first ring.

"Doctor, don't be alarmed. My son isn't sick. I'm not going to spoil your New Year's Eve." He lowered his voice. "Your wife just went up to Wells's apartment with a suitcase in her hand. It's nothing new. She visits him regularly every Saturday and Sunday afternoons. But New Year's Eve! Don't feel bad, though. Remember what Kipling said: 'A woman is only a woman but a good cigar is a smoke.'"

"I wouldn't know. I never use them," said Jim.

"Still in training, huh? Well, have a happy New Year and don't do anything I wouldn't do."

"What's left?" said Jim and hung up.

I hope his wife is cheating on him in heaven, he said to himself, screwing some lecherous angel whose slowly beating wings cool her during the sexual act so that unconsumed by the celestial passion, she is ready for an infinity of encores. Secret agent Roach, unsolicited spy, a worthy shadower of Annie Laurie! It's no use being too hard on him, though. The bastard is probably outraged at the way she is treating his pediatrician.

Jim picked up the evening *Post,* but the words had no meaning for him. After failing to concentrate for a few minutes, he telephoned Trudy.

"Annie Laurie is spending the night with Wells. I just got the news from my peeping Tom. I suppose you have a date for this evening."

"Of course I do," said Trudy. "With you."

"Then let's make it for this New Year's Eve and every New Year's Eve hereafter. And dress up. We're going to the Waldorf."

"Jimmy! You'll never get reservations this late."

"We'll see."

He rang up one of the managers of the hotel whose son's life he had saved ten years before by making a slick diagnosis of acute retrocecal appendicitis. There was no difficulty in getting a table. The man had an excellent memory. Trudy looked radiant in a low cut white evening gown, a mature Jenny Velvet from the neck down. After the headwaiter had ushered them to their table, she said,

"One of the reasons I like you is that you still look like a thug even in evening clothes. I once knew a man who would have seemed well-dressed disguised as a chimney sweep. He's the one who gave me the pictures. He's dead now."

"Then I don't have to kill him."

She reached across the table and squeezed his hand. "You already have."

When Guy Lombardo crossed the bandstand, Jim said, "I hope he plays either a gavotte or a minuet; that's what they were doing the last time I danced."

"Oh, Jimmy, nobody expects you to do the funky Broadway or the boog-a-loog. He will play lots of old-fashioned fox trots. You'll see."

She was right. They took possession of a square yard of the crowded floor, held each other tightly, and made rhythmic movements with their feet, which, while not as spectacular as those once achieved by Nijinsky and Lydia Lopokova in *Spectre de la Rose,* brought them a degree of intimacy the Russian dancers had never attained. When they returned to their table Jim gave her a full report on what had taken place at the meeting of the joint conference committee. Then they drank a bottle of champagne. At midnight, when the band played

"Auld Lang Syne," they kissed each other. She reminded herself that she was fifty years old and unmarried, and had never before been kissed openly by a healthy man. There were only memories of assignations kept secret to preserve the good name of the British Foreign Service and heart-breaking nights spent alone nursing a frail and dying lover. She prayed that a day would soon come when everyone would acknowledge that this wonderful mountain of muscle belonged to her. Then if people asked her where she was going to spend her vacation, she could truthfully say to herself if not to them—on Mt. Keats or vice versa.

When they reached the door of her apartment at three in the morning, she said,

"Won't you come in? Your wife is going to be out all night."

He shook his head. "I'm afraid I would only botch things up. Maybe I'll have more confidence after the divorce. The spirit is willing but the flesh is weak."

As he took her in his arms and kissed her good night he felt the stirrings of desire for the first time in years. But after a moment her lips, which until then had been soft and exciting, suddenly seemed to turn hard. He realized that he was kissing her teeth. She was laughing. She watched him as he stepped back and buttoned his overcoat.

"You've got everything reversed," she said. "Your flesh is willing but your spirit is weak. All right, Jimmy, I can wait. I've been chaste longer than you."

Annie Laurie returned home at four o'clock New Year's afternoon. For the next two days she was particularly aloof. Then one evening at six she walked into the apartment glowing with happiness.

"Can't you put that paper away for one minute," she said to Jim. "Or maybe you're not interested in what I am going to tell you." She took off her coat and sat down. "I'm pregnant."

Jim dropped his paper. "You're out of your mind. It's impossible."

"Is it? Dr. Akt says I am and he is Director of the Department of Obstetrics, and president of the medical board, isn't he? He just told me that any woman who has an ovary, a tube, and a uterus can become pregnant." She laughed bitterly. "You must have been shooting blanks all those years. There's nothing wrong with me. I'm a normal woman. I'm going to have a baby."

She went into the kitchen and returned with two drinks. "You are not going to make any trouble about the divorce, are you?"

"No trouble at all," said Jim.

She laughed. "I'm not claiming that this is an immaculate conception. The poor baby was conceived in sin. That's not his fault, though. You know all about it, including who the father is." She patted his cheek. "Don't feel bad. You and I really haven't been married for years. Just the same, I haven't forgotten the nice things you did for me in the early days. I'm just swapping one pediatrician for another. It isn't as if I were going outside your specialty to find a new husband." A dreamy look came into her eyes. "He doesn't know that he is going to be a father. I told you first for old times' sake. We did have fun in the beginning, didn't we? I think it was the lack of money and the snoring that finally did our marriage in. I can hear you through two closed doors. I won't need any alimony. He can support a wife and child quite nicely. And I am bringing him two income-tax exemptions and a dowry."

"What do you mean, a dowry?"

"Oh, you know about most of it. You must have guessed the rest. It's the one thing I'm ashamed of. Yes, I gave him the virus killer or what I thought was the virus killer, but not because I hated you or loved him. I gave it to him for thirty-five thousand dollars. With my family history I had to. Some women have a family history of insanity or diabetes. Mine is poverty. I begged you to cash in on the virus killer, remember? When you refused, that was the end. There went my last chance for financial security. I had to try to get a little nest egg together on my own if you wouldn't do it for me, didn't I? You understand. Please forgive me."

"Of course I'll forgive you. You didn't do me any harm. You didn't get the virus killer. As a matter of fact, the botched-up burglary knocked my only rival out of the running. If I get the job, I will owe it to you."

Tears came to Annie Laurie's eyes. "You're all right, Jim."

The following evening the tears had become torrential. When he came home he found her sobbing on the sofa. He put his hand on her shoulder and asked,

"What's the matter? Aren't you pregnant after all?"

"I'm pregnant. And I'm going to stay pregnant until I have a big beautiful baby later this year." She looked up at Jim. "He says I have to have an abortion. He's not going to marry me."

Jim sat down slowly. "That's just his first reaction. You must have thrown him into a state of shock. One minute he is a carefree bachelor, the next you tell him he has a wife and family on his hands. What did you expect him to say? Give him time. He'll change his mind."

She dried her eyes and looked at him again. "Do you really think he will marry me?"

Jim gave her a wicked smile. "I guarantee it."

The next morning he sat down in Wells's consultation room long before the first patient was scheduled to appear.

"I hope you won't consider me old-fashioned," he said to his young colleague. "I didn't say anything while you were screwing my wife. That's not old-fashioned, is it? But I have certain family rules. One of them is this: Anyone who gets my wife pregnant has to marry her. You got her pregnant. You'll have to marry her."

"Can you prove I am the father?" asked Wells. "You're the big Rh-and-blood-group man. Sure, anybody can prove nonpaternity. But you know damn well that it is impossible to prove paternity. I am group A, Rh positive like thirty-five percent of the population. There's not a test in the world that can show that I'm the father."

"You're the father, all right. Annie Laurie is not a tramp. But I'm not interested in blood groups. And the two million readers of the *Daily News* won't be interested in them either. They will be impressed by the juicy testimony of your apartment-house superintendent, and the pictures of the sucker who went after the triple crown and fell on his face, the sucker who tried to steal a senior colleague's wife, position, and virus killer and ended up with nothing but a woman he didn't want. You'll have to marry Annie Laurie, my boy."

"Why? Don't you have enough money for an abortion? You'll get professional courtesy."

Jim looked at his big fists. "I do now. But I feel guilty. I blame myself for some of this mess. The day Roach told me that my wife was visiting you I should have gone to your apartment and beaten your brains out. I didn't because I'm not a violent man. But if Annie Laurie doesn't file for a divorce within a week—and I think she will— and if you don't marry her the day after she gets it, I am going down to the district attorney with Captain Prince's report and have you prosecuted for grand larceny."

"Do you think you can make it stick?" asked Wells with a smile.

Jim noticed that under the tan he was a trifle pale. "I think so, especially if Annie Laurie turns state's evidence and testifies that you gave her thirty-five thousand dollars to open the refrigerator. I have a feeling she will. A woman scorned, you know."

"I don't think you will go through with this," said Wells after a moment. "You're an old Adams buff and this would give the hospital a black eye."

Jim laughed. "The trustees would like to give you one. You're not an Adams man. But I'm not vindictive. I don't want you to go to jail. I just want to ruin you. If I am made director of Pediatrics, the first thing I will do will be to kick you off the service, with the blessings of the board of trustees, I might add. Then I will go up to the Medical Center and tell Professor Choate, whom I have known since we went to medical school together, Dr. Locke, whom I played football against in college, and Mr. Wright, a wonderful and very powerful old trustee, all the details of the burglary that did not appear in the newspapers. Do you think that you will ever get a job at the Medical Center after that? Or an affiliation with any other hospital in Manhattan? The press will show you up not only as a crook but a dumb crook, a doctor willing to pay thirty-five thousand dollars for the chance to steal a little ordinary salt solution. Where will you send your private patients if you don't have any hospital connections? To some grubby little sanitarium in Queens? Your practice will just melt away."

"All right, all right!" said Wells. "I get the picture." He seemed a little rattled. "What will you do for me if I marry Ann?"

"The day you marry her I will send you the original of Captain Prince's report as a wedding present. That may not seem like much considering the thousands of Xerox copies I can have made. But with it will go my word that I will drop this matter. Then I will tell Mr. Guthrie and Mr. Crunch that I want you to stay on the service, that I feel I can reform you. In addition, I will encourage you to send your private patients to Adams. The more you send in, the fewer the empty beds. Finally, there will be no publicity about the incident. If I am asked about it, I will play dumb. You will get not only a beautiful wife with whom you are sexually compatible but a child, your own child. In pediatrics a family is good for business. Your practice will flourish. Wells, you have to face reality. If you screw enough women, even married women, eventually you will get hooked. What do you say?"

Wells hesitated but not for long. "I don't suppose you would shake hands with me on this."

"If it's the conclusion of a deal, sure."

"It's the conclusion of a deal."

They stood up and shook hands.

"There's one final request," said Jim. "Please don't tell Annie Laurie that I was here."

Wells smiled. "I'm always willing to do anything that makes me look good."

They walked to the door.

"For some time now," said Wells, "I've been wondering whether there wasn't another woman involved in this case."

"What's the matter," said Jim, "didn't you think I was young enough?"

Wells shook his head. "I didn't think you were smart enough."

When Jim returned home that evening, the drinks were on the living room table. Annie Laurie threw her arms around him and kissed him on the cheek.

"Everything turned out just as you prophesied. He's going to marry me the day after I get the divorce. You were right. All that stuff he told me yesterday was just the first reaction of a confirmed bachelor thrown into a panic. Thank you for cheering me up. I'm taking the plane the day after tomorrow."

Jim reached into his pocket and handed her a check for a thousand dollars. Her eyes widened as she took it.

"What's this for?" she asked.

"For breakfast in bed."

18

ON SUNDAY evening January the twentieth Clair Crunch, the eleven-year-old daughter of the chairman of the board, complained of numbness and pain in her right leg. Her mother rubbed it with scented bath oil. Her father was deeply upset. This man who could stand great physical suffering himself was thrown into a panicky rage at the thought of anything hurting his fairy princess. He called her that in part because of her shoulder-covering golden hair and delicate features but principally because he loved her so much. She was the youngest of his five children. The others were boys. The next morning she had a temperature of a hundred and three. Mrs. Crunch called Dr. Syms, a mild, middle-aged pediatrician from another hospital who had taken care of her daughter since the day of her birth. When her husband had become chairman of the board five years previously, she had refused to switch to a member of the Adams staff. Syms, she knew, though not brilliant, was conscientious and faithful. Besides, the whole thing was ridiculous. Clair saw a doctor once a year for a school examination.

He went over her thoroughly, performing a few simple neurological tests. Her neck was stiff, her right leg weak. Just as he finished she had a short convulsion. The maid remained with her while he ushered the parents into the hall.

"She's a sick girl," he said. "She should be in the hospital."

"You're on the courtesy staff. You have private privileges at Adams. Put her in," said Crunch. "But what has she got?"

"Acute encephalitis," answered Dr. Syms.

"What does that mean?"

"An inflammation of the brain."

"Well, don't do a lot of painful tests on her when you get her to the hospital," said Crunch gruffly.

The ambulance brought her to Adams within an hour. That afternoon the chief resident performed a lumbar puncture. The protein and white cells in the spinal fluid were somewhat elevated. That was all. When Syms came to Adams at eight o'clock the following morning, the Crunches were sitting by their daughter's bedside looking as if they had not slept all night. Clair was much worse. Her temperature was a hundred and five and she was having frequent, generalized convulsions. Her right leg was paralyzed. She was hallucinating. Syms took the parents aside.

"The protein and white cells in her spinal fluid were slightly elevated. And it was water-clear. That is the picture in viral encephalitis. But the white cells in her blood are greatly elevated, over twenty-five thousand, three times the normal. That doesn't usually go with a viral infection. I feel we should have a second opinion."

"Get the best man in town," said Crunch.

"The most famous clinician in town is Backman of Mt. Sinai," said Syms. "He is seventy-five and was trained in the great days of the free wards, when a lowly intern would have fifty patients under his care. He has seen everything and knows everything. The only trouble is that he is apt to be brusque and even rude at times."

"I've heard of him. Who am I to complain?" said Crunch. "I am not noted for my gentle diplomacy, am I? Get him."

Promptly at ten Backman marched up to the nurses' station on the seventh floor. He was a doctor of the old school who believed in getting to the patient fast. Not for him was the stratagem of the distant appointment often employed by some of his colleagues to impress their patients. His wife had reported an almost unbelievable conversation to him after returning from a consultation with an orthopedist who was treating her for a minor back problem. The secretary was supposed to have said to someone over the telephone, "We can see you at eleven A.M. three weeks from tomorrow." There had been a long pause. Then she had exclaimed, "Really! He actually threatens to break your lease because you moan and scream all night? Well, why didn't you tell me that in the first place, my dear lady?" After going through her appointment book, she announced, "In that case we will of course see you sooner. Let's make it *one* week from tomorrow." Backman realized that his wife would resort to any exaggeration to improve a story. Nevertheless, this time her tale had the familiar ring of truth. The device of the distant appointment had been responsible for the rapid rise of more than one of his medical friends. If an ophthalmologist, an eye man, for instance, could see to it that enough women said, "I couldn't get an appointment with him for three months and I'm his wife's best friend!" or better still, "He's not taking any new patients until next August," his success was practically assured. People tended to value that which was hard to get. Obviously, a specialist who could not see you for three months was a better doctor than one who could not see you for two. The patients not only put up with these distant appointments, they boasted about them. Backman thought back to an anecdote he had heard many years before. When Radio City was completed, it was said that the architect had taken John D. Rockefeller on a tour of the huge complex. Halfway through, the man said, "Now I would like to show you your office. I think you will find it very impressive." Rockefeller looked at him in amazement and said, "Whom would I want to impress?" That was exactly the way Backman felt. Whom would he want to impress? Not for him was the distant appointment. He saw the patient fast.

He knew quite well that in New York the legends of his magic diagnoses were just as fresh as they had been at any time during the past half century. With a yearning he could not suppress, his mind returned to the days when he had been a young doctor, especially to the first rounds of the season when he met the rookie interns. On these occasions he would invariably enter the ward with a small notebook in his left hand and a bright red ribbon tied to the thumb of his right. Soon the house staff would be spellbound by the brilliance of his analyses, the keenness of his diagnoses, and his encyclopedic knowledge of the medical literature. As he finished with each little patient, he would write something in his memo book. The red ribbon never left his finger, even when he put on the glove for a rectal examination. In the end, he would explain to the interns that he used the little book to help him remember the condition of each child. Then he would wait. Inevitably one of the more gullible interns would ask, "Sir, what is the red ribbon for?" To which Backman would reply, "To remind me to look in the book." Ah, those were the days of the great eccentrics, the great actors, the great medical magicians! If a man combined the qualities of all three, maybe someday he would become a great diagnostician. Yes, those were the days when the hospital was run by brain power, not by steel and human machines. True, medicine was a thousand times greater today, but still . . . !

Backman stood at the nurses' station, tall and gaunt, his back still ramrod straight, his bearing military. He wore a black broadcloth suit which after all these years had acquired a faint rusty sheen in bright sunlight. Stretching between the lower pockets of his vest was a gold chain. Like the railroad conductors of yesteryear, he had never worn a wristwatch. The sartorial climax of his outfit was an incredibly high, stiff white collar whose half-inch vertical slit mercilessly gripped his necktie knot. It was in fact an Arrow Collar Belmont, and nothing like it had been seen in New York in over forty years. The assistant nursing supervisor looked at him in awe and astonishment. What a pity it was, she said to herself, that Miss Starr was not here to see this remarkable man. But she was helping Dr. Keats examine a very sick boy and nothing took precedence over Dr. Keats.

Dr. Syms and the Crunches hurried along the corridor to the nurses' station. Backman looked down at Joe Crunch and said severely,

"Why do you need me? You have Syms. I'm just an old-fashioned pediatrician from the sidewalks of New York."

Molly Crunch smiled sadly. "That's exactly what we want. We are old-fashioned. We are New Yorkers. And we are practically of the same generation as you."

Backman took the forty-five-year-old woman's hand, patted it gently, and said, "I love to be flattered."

It took him only a few minutes to read through the chart. The child's illness was only a day and a half old and her past history was uneventful. Guided by Dr. Syms and the Crunches, he led the way to Clair's room. Two nurses stood motionless by the bedside. The patient seemed to be totally possessed by fear. Her mouth was twisted, her eyes fixed on some unimaginable horror. But Backman seemed interested only in an area of skin two inches above her right ankle. The moment he picked up her leg, the two nurses could tell that he knew the diagnosis. All they were able to see were two healed small puncture marks. His examination was brief, almost perfunctory. But he scrubbed his hands for a long time in the sink at the other end of the spacious private room and searched them carefully for cuts and abrasions after they were dry.

"Nurse, please let me have a glass of water," he said, watching Clair closely.

The effect that this request had upon the child was electrifying. She thrashed at the bed with her arms and good leg, her eyes wild and pleading. He took the glass, held it a foot from her lips and said,

"Drink this."

Clair made a strangled, crowing noise and stopped breathing. Although her chest heaved, she could get no oxygen into her lungs. Soon she turned blue. With clawed hands she reached out for air.

"Spasm of the glottis," said Backman to Syms coldly. "It's a text-book case."

For an interminable minute she fought the spasm. Then it relaxed and she could breathe once more.

"She almost died!" whispered Mrs. Crunch.

It would have been better if she had, Backman thought. Then she would have been spared the hideous suffering of the next few days. He pointed to the corridor. They all followed him.

As soon as the door closed he said, "Your daughter has rabies, one of the oldest of the recorded diseases. Aristotle described it twenty-three hundred years ago. When I was a boy, people called it hydrophobia, dread of water. You just saw what happened when I showed her the glass. When was she bitten, Mr. Crunch?"

The chairman of the board stood silent, his eyes as vacant as if he were under a spell.

"Mr. Crunch," repeated Backman harshly, "do you deny that she was bitten? I just saw the marks on her leg."

Joe Crunch's eyes slowly focused on Backman's chest. "Over four months ago. That's too far in the past for there to be any connection, isn't it?" he begged.

"I'm afraid not," said Backman, sighing. He sighed about once a year. "The incubation period may be as long as six months, and in rare instances even a year."

"It was such a small bite," said Molly Crunch. "After a few weeks we thought we were in the clear. When Clair got sick the other day, I remembered the dog for a moment. But only for a moment. We must have believed that if we pushed the connection from our minds it would go away."

"It never went away," said Backman. "How many injections against rabies did she have?"

"None," said Joe Crunch. "I wouldn't let them hurt her." He

turned toward Dr. Syms and added apologetically, "You were on vacation."

"Is there any chance that our little girl might recover?" asked Molly Crunch.

"No," replied Backman. "Rabies is an ancient disease, yet I know of only one patient who ever recovered—Hattwick's case—and that boy had received fourteen antirabies injections after he was bitten."

"I killed her," said Joe Crunch. He walked back to his daughter's room muttering, "It's perfectly simple. I killed her."

"This will kill him, too," said his wife. She turned to Backman. "What causes rabies, Doctor?"

Backman gave a bitter laugh. "What causes everything today? A virus. Only this one is neurotropic. It gets into the nervous system and never lets go."

He looked at Syms. "It's secreted in the patient's saliva. So tell the nurses to protect themselves."

For the second time he took Molly Crunch's hand and patted it. "She must have been a beautiful girl."

Then he walked down the corridor, ramrod straight like those Junker officers at the turn of the century who were said to have worn corsets under their beautiful uniforms.

Four and a half months before, on a mild morning early in September, Molly Crunch was sitting on a bench in Central Park watching her daughter roller skate on the concrete path in front of her. Walking slowly from the opposite direction was a big, black Labrador retriever. As Clair came abreast of him, he snapped at her right leg just above the ankle. She skated to the grass trying to hold back her tears and sat down. A girl in her mid-twenties ran up and said to Molly, who was patting her daughter's head,

"Oh, I'm so sorry. The noise of the roller skates must have frightened him." She turned to the dog. "Schweitzer, sit!" He sat on the grass as if nothing had happened. In her set it was considered a mark of sophistication to give a dog an unusual name. Her fiancé had called him Schweitzer because he had a big organ. Their friends thought this a terribly clever inside joke. The yahoos outside would never know that Albert Schweitzer was an accomplished organist.

She bent over the child's leg. "It doesn't look like much."

"The skin is broken," said Molly. "Has the dog received his rabies shots?"

"Yes, indeed, and distemper, too. Everything."

She did not mention that Schweitzer had received his only anti-rabies inoculation when he was ten months old. He was ten years now.

Molly said, "Will you please let me have your name and address?"

The girl wrote them on a card and handed it to her. "My phone number is there, too. It's unlisted."

"And you *will* take your dog to the vet, won't you?"

"The first thing tomorrow. May I have your name and address?"

Molly wrote them down for her.

Since Dr. Syms was away, she took her daughter to the Adams emergency room. The resident found two small, rather superficial puncture wounds two inches above her right ankle. He cleaned them meticulously, poured Zephiran over them, and gave the child an injection of tetanus toxoid. Then he rang up the Bureau of Animal Bites of the New York City Department of Health and let them have the required information.

The telephone was ringing when Schweitzer and the girl entered her apartment. The call was from her fiancé in Savannah, who had been stricken with acute appendicitis just before he was about to leave for New York. He was going to be operated upon early that evening. Unless she came down to look after him, he felt sure that he would die of complications. He was such a baby, she said to herself. The handsome hypochondriac! But she could not refuse. The week they had spent together in New Hampshire early in August had been too good.

Schweitzer had had a good time, too, roaming through the woods and fields, unsupervised and uncared for. Once to his astonishment a skunk had barred his way, and then, instead of spraying him with its foul secretion, had sprung forward and bitten him in the neck. The dog had brushed it to the ground with a forepaw and, seizing it by the neck with his jaws, had shaken it until it was dead. The skunk's attack was precipitated not by courage but by rabies, a disease quite prevalent among the species. The little animal never knew how fortunate it was to have been given the quick, merciful death of a mauling instead of the slow, cruel one of this most hideous of sicknesses. The lovers never discovered the tiny wound in Schweitzer's neck. They fed him regularly and copiously and ignored him. There was too much to be discovered in each other.

The girl was thinking of the New Hampshire week when she put down the telephone. Suddenly she remembered the child her dog had bitten. She sat at her desk and wrote a letter to Molly Crunch explaining that she was going down South to visit her fiancé, who was about to have an emergency operation. As soon as she reached her destination, she promised to take Schweitzer to a vet. If there was anything wrong with him, she would telephone New York at once. In the meantime, Mrs. Crunch was not to worry. The dog was perfectly healthy.

At six o'clock the following morning she drove down to Savannah in her Buick sedan with the big Labrador retriever in the seat next to her. At eleven o'clock a policeman rang her bell on and off for five minutes. When there was no answer, he slipped a paper under the door. It was a notice from the Department of Health ordering her to deliver a biting animal for examination within four days. The girl was given a choice. She could have the animal looked at by a private veterinarian at her own expense or by a veterinarian of the Department of Health free of charge. The address of the Manhattan ASPCA was included. If the animal was found not to be sick, she would be requested to bring it in for a final examination ten days from the date of the bite.

For five months the notice rested unread on the floor of her apartment. The girl reached her destination, the Savannah General Hospital, on time, but as a patient not a visitor. The first night she spent in a quiet and luxurious motel. But she got little sleep. From nine in the evening until six the next morning Schweitzer growled and howled and snapped at flies that were not there. Everyone was glad to see them go. On the last leg of the journey the dog, crouched on the seat next to her, grew constantly more restless. As they entered the outskirts of the city, he threw himself against her in one mighty convulsive movement. The wheel spun and the automobile careened across the road and into a concrete abutment. The unlocked door on the passenger side flew open and Schweitzer was thrown against a tree. He died instantly. Within three minutes the state troopers were there. They pulled the unconscious girl out of the smoldering car and laid her gently on the grass. At the hospital a team of physicians and surgeons discovered that she had a fractured skull, a fractured pelvis, and a compound fracture of the femur.

After two days she regained consciousness but with no memory of the accident. Three months later her parents took her to their home in a suburb of Chicago to convalesce. Schweitzer's body was disposed of by the Sanitation Department of the City of Savannah. Nobody suspected that he had rabies with Negri bodies in the brain and virus in the saliva.

Two weeks after Clair had been bitten, the New York City Police Department had telephoned Mr. Crunch. The girl had not taken her dog to a vet. She was not at home. Crunch laughed and read the sergeant the letter. But that afternoon he sent his head of security to interview the superintendent of her apartment house on Manhattan's upper East Side. He learned that she had been a model tenant and had lived there with the dog for five years. The following afternoon Joe and Molly went to the Medical Center to consult a nationally known authority on rabies. He listened to the facts and read the letter. Then he wiped his glasses to gain a little time and said,

"This is a tough case. I am almost tempted to say that you have to make the decision yourself. You see, if the dog had rabies, there is no guarantee that injections begun sixteen days after the bite instead of immediately would prevent the disease. Nevertheless, I recommend that your daughter receive twenty daily injections of the vaccine followed by boosters ten and twenty days after the completion of the course."

"Is there a chance that the injections themselves might cause permanent damage?" asked Molly.

The expert shook his head. "You're thinking of the old Semple vaccine. That did cause permanent paralysis. But the newer duck-embryo vaccine is relatively harmless."

"Where would these twenty-two injections be given?" asked Joe.

"Under the skin of the abdomen."

Joe winced. "Are they painful?"

"I'm afraid they are," the doctor replied.

"Is it true, Doctor," continued Joe, "that there has not been a case of rabies in New York City in twenty years?"

"It's true, and we want to keep it that way."

Joe hesitated. "If you will bear with us, Doctor, Mrs. Crunch and I would like to talk this over."

Clair never received the preventive inoculations against rabies.

Backman would have been interested in hearing of Schweitzer's encounter with the skunk, his strange behavior on the trip to Savannah, and his violent death. But not inordinately so. The old man was always so sure of his diagnoses. As he walked away from Clair's room he wanted only to drive the case from his mind. Ordinarily he was not affected by fatal illness. But this was so unnecessary. Striding down the corridor as if to the music of a military band, he saw Jim and Trudy standing by the bedside of a boy whose neck was arched backward on the mattress. He poked his head through the doorway.

"What's the cause of the meningitis, Jim?" he asked.

Trudy looked at him in amazement.

"The herpes-simplex virus, sir," replied Jim.

Backman shook his head. "Aren't you a law-and-order man? I refer to the law of probabilities and the scientific order it brings. Herpes meningitis is very rare, improbable, in fact. Don't forget good old meningococcal meningitis." He turned toward Trudy. "And who is the beautiful lady?"

"I'm sorry," said Jim. "Miss Starr."

Backman bowed from the hips. His back remained stiff. "Jim was afraid to introduce me because he knows that I am a better diagnostician than he." He surveyed her buxom beauty with a connoisseur's eyes. "After meeting you I think I will go home and ask my wife for a divorce. The only thing that is holding me back is that she would gladly give it to me. After being married to me for fifty years she will want to try someone else."

"Not if you look at her the way you are looking at me now," said Trudy.

A smile creased Backman's pale face. He smiled about once a year. "By George, I think I'll try it."

He walked away, his military air enhanced by the clicking of his metal-tipped heels on the tile floor.

"Who is that wonderful man?" asked Trudy.

"The legendary Dr. Backman," answered Jim. He told her a little about him.

"Is he really a better diagnostician than you?"

"Much better."

"Impossible," said Trudy.

At eight that morning Jim had received a call from Mr. Roach. His son had been vomiting since early the previous day. At first the superintendent had thought that it was the one-day stomach flu. But now the boy's temperature was a hundred and four and he could not be roused. Jim met the Roaches in the Adams emergency room. The child was comatose, his neck rigid, and the lower portion of his face covered with fever blisters. No telltale petechiae, those tiny hemorrhages which are the hallmark of meningococcal meningitis, could be found anywhere on his skin or mucous membranes. Jim spoke to Roach in the waiting room.

"Your boy has meningitis and he is very sick. It can be a bacterial meningitis, that is one caused by a germ, or a viral meningitis. I think it is a meningitis caused by the virus in those fever blisters, the herpes-simplex virus. I'll have the blood count any minute now. If it is high, say thirty thousand, it's probably a bacterial meningitis. If it is low, say six thousand, it is probably a viral meningitis. As soon as we can get everything set up in the examining room, we are going to do a spinal tap. That will clinch the diagnosis."

A quarter of an hour before Backman poked his head into the doorway of the boy's room the blood count was handed to Jim. He left Trudy with the patient and sought out the superintendent.

"Mr. Roach, the blood count is fifty-nine hundred. I think your boy has a meningo-encephalitis caused by the herpes-simplex virus."

"Are there drugs for it?" asked Roach.

"None that really work."

A crafty look came over Roach's face. "I hear from the grapevine that you have a drug that kills viruses. Isn't my son sick enough for it?"

"He's sick enough, all right."

"I've got a lot of money salted away. It's all yours. And I'll say whatever you want on the witness stand when I testify for you at your divorce proceedings."

Jim looked at the super somberly. This vulgar man disgusted him. "I don't want your money." He did not mention that his divorce would soon be final. "I'll do it for nothing."

"Do I have your word on it?" asked Roach.

"I just told you that I'd do it," snapped Jim.

He went back to the boy's room and asked Trudy to go to her apartment and get the virus killer for him. She hurried to her office, threw her overcoat over her uniform, and was back in twenty minutes.

"I just now put it in the refrigerator in the examining room," she said breathlessly. "The last little Indian!"

"Big Indian," said Jim.

He looked up. Joe Crunch was standing in the doorway. Jim took off his isolation gown and walked into the corridor in his shirtsleeves.

"Dr. Backman has just told Mrs. Crunch and me that our daughter has rabies," said Crunch. "And that it is a uniformly fatal disease. I learned a moment ago from my wife that it is caused by a virus." He looked up at Jim pleadingly. "What can we do to persuade you to give the last dose of the virus killer to our little girl?"

Jim sighed. "I hate to break your heart, but I can't let her have it. I've already promised to give it to that desperately ill boy in there. You think I have a choice. I don't. I have to do everything in my power for every one of my patients. I can't withhold a life-saving remedy from one of them in order to give it to a child I have never seen even though she may deserve it more. I don't suppose I should have given half of my dwindling supply to Professor Choate for analysis, but I never imagined I would be in a spot like this. You probably regard me as an executioner. If I am, I'm an unwilling one. I can only ask you to forgive me."

"Is there nothing you can do for Clair, nothing?" asked Crunch.

Jim shook his head. "No one recovers from rabies."

Crunch threw up his hands and walked away. The little giant looked very little indeed. But he would not give up. He used the telephone at the nurses' station to ask Dummer to come to the seventh floor as soon as possible. The Director of Pediatrics was there in five minutes. Crunch told him everything about the case, including his conversation with Jim.

"What I would like you to do," he concluded, "is to use medical arguments to make Dr. Keats change his mind. For instance, the way things now stand my daughter has no chance at all of recovering. If that boy down the corridor has a fifty percent chance of recovering, Dr. Keats should use the virus killer on Clair, shouldn't he?"

"I'll see what I can do," said Dummer.

He put on a gown, walked into the room where Jim and Trudy were sitting by the bedside, and beckoned him to the far corner.

"Are you out of your mind!" exclaimed Dummer. "You'll never get that job if you refuse to give your virus killer to the daughter of the chairman of the board of trustees. You must be the most naive man in Adams. Don't you want to be the director of Pediatrics? Then why did you apply? Sure, I did everything in my power to push Bridge Wells ahead. But since he fell on his face, I'll have to be satisfied with someone else. I've decided that I don't want to see an outsider take over my job. And take over he will if you don't lapse back into sanity. I admit that I've never been a friend of yours, but I would prefer the devil I know to the university hospital devil I don't. There is another thing. I would like Crunch to think well of me. The way things stand now he will always feel I have been harboring an idiot on my staff."

"I want the job," said Jim, "but I also want to sleep at night. I am pledged to give the virus killer to this boy. He is my patient and I am not going to abandon him."

Dummer shrugged. "It's not only Clair's funeral. It's yours."

He walked along the corridor until he came up to Joe Crunch standing in front of his daughter's door.

"I couldn't budge him. He's a mule," said Dummer.

Seated at the boy's bedside, Trudy looked up at Jim, who was standing at the far end of the room watching his chief walk away.

"I should have gone into pro football instead of medicine," he said.

"No, you shouldn't," she said. "You did the right thing, the only thing. You're an old-fashioned straight arrow and a straight arrow can't bend. It's simply terrible about that little girl, but on the other hand you can't let the boy die either. As far as the salary goes, don't worry about it. I can always sell a few pictures."

Jim went up to her and patted her head. "I'm not used to having a woman stick up for me. You know, Trudy, I would kiss your hands if there weren't so much infection in this room."

He went to the telephone and asked the page operator to get Dr. Cheecheecastanango at once. He did this first because he liked to hear the name over the loudspeakers, and second because he had promised the young doctor to call him before he used the virus killer.

José appeared in less than a minute. He listened attentively as Jim presented the case, demonstrated the stiff neck, and discussed the facial herpes.

"How many lumbar punctures have you done?" asked Jim.

"About thirty, sir, all in Argentina."

"Would you like to do this one?"

José bowed.

"What do you think the spinal fluid will be like?" asked Jim.

"Clear, with about fifty cells, all lymphocytes."

Jim nodded. "The boy is as stiff as a board. I'd better bend him for the tap."

Trudy had put three of her best nurses in the examining room. The equipment was ready. Gowned and wearing sterile rubber gloves, José slipped the needle into the spinal canal with ease. Everyone leaned forward as he pulled out the stylet. Turbid fluid squirted into the test tube.

"Jeez!" exclaimed Jim. "It's an old-fashioned bacterial meningitis!"

As soon as the procedure was completed José took the tube and hurried to the laboratory to get the technicians to do an immediate cell count and culture on the spinal fluid. Jim helped Trudy and one of her nurses wheel the boy back to his room on a stretcher. He was in a coma. Twenty minutes later José threw on an isolation gown and burst into the room with the report.

"There are eight thousand nine hundred cells in the spinal fluid, no lymphocytes. And the girls have picked up typical, biscuit-shaped, gram-negative diplococci. The culture won't be ready until tomorrow, but they all are sure, including the head technician, that the organisms are meningococci."

"Start him right away on four hundred milligrams of ampicillin per kilogram a day intravenously," said Jim. "We'll switch to twelve million units of penicillin tomorrow when the culture confirms the preliminary laboratory diagnosis."

"Why do you think the blood count was so low, sir?"

"I don't know. Maybe because of bone marrow suppression due to an overwhelming infection," answered Jim.

José hurried from the room.

"How could Dr. Backman make the correct diagnosis just by looking through the doorway?" asked Trudy.

"Well," said Jim, "when he saw that the boy's neck was so stiff that it was arched back like a bow, he figured that he had meningitis. Second, he knows that herpes-simplex meningoencephalitis is very rare. His law of probabilities, remember? Third, he reached back into his memory bank and recalled that many of his patients with meningococcal meningitis had fever blisters. It's not uncommon in that disease, you know. And fourth and most important, he's smart."

Trudy gave him a maternal smile. "When you are seventy-five, you will be just as smart as he."

Jim laughed, took off his isolation gown, and put on his white coat. He found Roach in the waiting room.

"Your son does not have a viral meningitis. He has a meningococcal meningitis. The virus killer wouldn't help him at all, but we have antibiotics that will."

"Do you think he has a chance, Doctor?"

"I think he's going to get well," said Jim.

Roach shook his head. "That wife of yours didn't deserve you."

Jim walked up to Clair's room, and, after knocking, opened the door. Everyone wore a surgical mask and an isolation gown. The Crunches took off theirs and came outside.

"I made the wrong diagnosis," said Jim. "The boy down the corridor does not have a viral infection. So if it's all right with you and Dr. Syms, I'll give your daughter the virus killer right now."

A silly look came over Crunch's hard face. He took his wife in his arms and kissed her. "Many happy wrong diagnoses, Molly."

Molly disengaged herself. "Doctor, do you think you'll be able to do for Clair what you did for Corky?"

"I don't know, Mrs. Crunch," said Jim. "I've never seen a case of rabies."

Joe had regained his confidence. "I'm not worried, Molly."

Jim walked to the nurses' station. In a few minutes he returned with Trudy. She was carrying the virus killer.

"I hope it hasn't lost its potency," he said.

"It hasn't lost its potency any more than you have," she replied. "Besides, I prayed over it every night."

They entered Clair's room and put on their masks and isolation gowns. José came in a moment later just as Jim was performing a complete physical and neurological examination on the child.

"Dr. Cheecheecastanango," he said, "the instant I puncture her skin she will probably go into a convulsion. Miss Starr will hold her arm. I want you to grab her so hard that she will not jar the needle out of the vein."

Trudy held out the tube while Jim removed the last three ml. of the virus killer with a sterile needle and syringe. As soon as he entered the vein, Clair went into a generalized convulsion, but Trudy and José gripped her so firmly that the injection was completed in a second. The instant the needle was removed, the convulsion stopped. Jim and Trudy sat by the bedside; José stood in the background. In a half hour the child seemed to fall into a deep natural sleep. In an hour her twisted mouth straightened. In an hour and a half her stiff neck became supple. In two hours she began to move her right leg. The room was now filled with gowned and masked nurses from all over the hospital who had come to see the miracle. Even the porter, a burly old man with six children, had donned a mask and gown. Trudy took the child's temperature. She announced that it was ninety-eight. A great silence settled over the room.

"In a few minutes I think the fairy princess is going to wake up," said Jim. "Please take off your gowns and masks. They would frighten the child out of her skin. Besides, you don't need them anymore."

All the gowns and masks were thrown into a pile. No one said a word. Five minutes later Clair yawned, sat up, and opened her eyes.

"Mommy," she cried, "where am I?"

Molly came forward and said, "In the hospital, dear. You were very sick."

Clair stretched. "I don't feel sick."

"Would you like a glass of cold water?" asked Jim.

Clair hesitated. Then she said, "Yes, I'm thirsty."

Trudy poured a glass of ice water from the metal carafe. The child drank it down eagerly. Everyone stood there spellbound. Suddenly out of the stillness the porter bellowed,

"This is the greatest thing I've seen since DiMaggio robbed Al Gionfriddo of a homer in the 1947 World Series!"

Trudy gave the man a withering look. "May I remind you that this is not Yankee Stadium."

Aha, said the porter to himself, she knows more about baseball than she lets on. It could have been Ebbets Field. But out loud he said contritely,

"I'm sorry, Miss Starr. I thought you were a Yankee fan."

"I'm a Dr. Keats fan," replied Trudy.

"So are we one and all," said Molly Crunch. She sounded like a character out of Dickens.

Jim began to feel embarrassed. "I'll be back at four," he said.

On the way out he passed close to José. "Don't you have to be somewhere?" he whispered.

"At a lecture," the resident replied. "But with your permission I'd rather stay with the patient."

Jim smiled. "Watch out. If you keep this up, you'll be a doctor before you know it."

Promptly at four he returned. Trudy and José were still there. Clair was sitting in a chair. Everyone else had left except the Crunches and the two special nurses. Jim ordered the child back to bed and examined her carefully. There was not a single abnormal finding.

"I just met Mr. Guthrie in the lobby," he said. "He told me that you go to dancing school. Will you show me a step?"

Clair did an eleven-year-old's version of an entrechat. Much to his surprise, she managed to land on her feet. Jim turned to the Crunches and said, "If it's all right with Dr. Syms, she can go home tomorrow."

"Dr. Syms is giving up practice and taking a full-time job out West," said Joe. "Will you be our children's doctor? There are five of them, but I won't ask for a wholesale rate."

"All right," said Jim. "I'll be your retail pediatrician."

Clair stepped up to him, her golden hair covering her shoulders. She smiled and a dimple appeared in her cheek. Eleven years old, he thought, and already a charmer and a flirt.

"Will I be all right when I grow up?"

"Certainly," said Jim.

"Will I be as beautiful as Miss Starr?"

An eleven-year-old charmer, Jim repeated to himself. He glanced at Trudy and then looked at Clair sternly. "Nobody will ever be as beautiful as Miss Starr. But you will be beautiful enough and you will marry a fairy tale prince."

"I don't want to marry a fairy tale prince. I want to marry a garbage man like my father or a football player like you."

Jim bent down and whispered, "I've got someone better for you."

She looked up eagerly.

"Corky Guthrie," he said.

She smiled and this time two dimples showed. "He's nice."

Jim walked out with Joe Crunch behind him. When they reached the corridor the chairman of the board said,

"Send me the bill tomorrow and don't spare the horses."

He passed his hand over his eyes. "I want you to believe this. You've got to believe it. I would have voted for you even if you hadn't given the virus killer to Clair." His hard face softened and tears came to his eyes. "You're a good man, Doctor," he said and went back to the room.

Trudy and José came out and strolled down the corridor with Jim.

The young doctor grinned. "I finally got to see one of your famous Juan Belmonte medical corridas. Two ears, the tail, and a hoof, sir!"

"Where were the residents?" asked Jim.

"At conferences, seminars, lectures, and demonstrations, or else making rounds with Dr. Dummer."

"Thank you for helping me," said Jim.

José bowed low. "Thank you for letting me watch from a front-row seat your *mano-a-mano* fight with death."

He bowed just as low to Trudy and walked away as if he were a young matador about to enter the arena.

She accompanied Jim to the elevator and smiled when he said, "I'll meet you at Oggi's at seven thirty."

He had been taking her out to dinner every night. Not once, however, did he go to her apartment or she to his. To do so, he feared, might tempt Wells to frame him with some evidence which he would shamelessly use to try to wriggle out of his agreement.

The following morning Jim sent the bill to Joe Crunch. Instead of a dollar figure he had his secretary type, "The King can do no wrong." Two days later he received a letter from the chairman of the board. As he held it in front of him he thought of the gracious note he had received from Tom Guthrie on a similar occasion. This one, he soon discovered, was quite different. It consisted of only one word, "Thanks." And it was signed, "Joseph, the First." He unfolded the check and stared at it. It was for thirty-five thousand dollars.

19

AT FOUR P.M. January twenty-fifth, 1974, Joe Crunch removed a big black cigar from its glass tube and, after snipping off the end, surveyed the six other trustees, the seven doctors, and the administrator who were assembled around the table in the council room for a special meeting of the joint conference committee. Then, to everyone's surprise, he put the cigar back in his pocket and walked up to Frank Ray. The Director of Radiology was coughing violently. He looked pale and sick.

"Why don't you take six months off?" asked Crunch. "On the house, of course. Lie on the sand in the Bahamas, sleep all afternoon, charge your batteries. After twenty-five years you deserve a semisabbatical."

He did not mention Hexter's reaction to the proposal earlier in the day.

"I see nothing wrong with it from the administrative point of view," Hexter had said. "The men in his department can carry on while he is away. But the vacation, as you so delicately put it, should be at his own expense, not ours. Personally, I wouldn't give him a cent. He didn't pick up that cancer from Adams. He got it from smoking two and a half packs of cigarettes a day."

Crunch had cocked his head to the side. "We pay you to be a heartless bastard, but there are times when you could use a cardiac transplant."

Ray looked up at the chairman of the board and shook his head. "Thanks, but there are a few things I have to clean up. Later there will be time enough to sleep."

Crunch forced a smile and returned to his seat at the head of the table. "You will remember," he said, "that at our last meeting I appointed Mr. Guthrie an ad hoc committee of one to report on suitable candidates for the position of director of Pediatrics. Tom."

There was a long silence while Guthrie riffled through some type-written pages. He looked up and said, "I mentioned the position to a few top-flight full-time men from the medical schools here. None of them were interested. First, they didn't want a part-time job. Second, they scoffed at the idea of leaving a university hospital to come to a voluntary one. Third, there was the question of salary." He skimmed through the report. "One of the older men put it best. Let's see. Oh, yes, here it is. I have it down almost verbatim. He said, 'The head of the Department of Pediatrics at Adams gets thirty-five thousand dollars a year on which to support his family. Two fourth-year residents who happen to be married to each other get thirty-six, plus a free room, free malpractice insurance, and fringe benefits. Why do you talk to me about a directorship? Why don't you make me an offer I can't refuse? Why don't you suggest that my wife and I become residents again?' "

Crunch looked at the trustees. "We were in the wrong line of work when we were kids. I used to get twenty a week for hauling garbage."

"I spoke to a few pediatricians in private practice who would have snapped up the position," continued Guthrie, "but they were not in the same league with Dr. Keats. The idea of taking a man who has never done anything for Adams and passing him over the head of a superior who has devoted thirty years of his life to our hospital is repugnant to me."

Crunch addressed himself to the doctors. "During the French Revolution some Jacobite hotheads sneaked across the German border, abducted two little princes of the blood who had sought refuge there, and murdered them. France was shocked. A prominent revolutionary went to Fouché and said, 'That was a crime.' The future minister of police fixed the man with his fishy eyes and replied, 'It was worse than a crime. It was a blunder.' When you voted to pass a shady kid like Wells over the head of an eminent pediatrician who has served the hospital for thirty years, what you did was worse than a crime. It was a blunder, because you opened the way for trustee interference in medical affairs. If you pull any more boners like this one, we are going to have to take over duties that once belonged to you. We feel that Dr. Keats is the man for the job. We are determined that he will be the next director of Pediatrics. Now why don't you go to the little conference room next door and see if you can't find a way out of your dilemma. We will wait here."

The doctors filed out rapidly. Scotti had his hand under Frank Ray's armpit. Within five minutes they returned.

"Have you come to a conclusion, Dr. Akt?" asked Crunch.

"Yes, we recommend that Dr. James Keats be made director of Pediatrics."

"An excellent choice," said Crunch. "And the vote?"

"Seven to nothing," replied Akt.

"Concensus, that's what I like to see, concensus," said the chairman of the board. "We will endorse your unanimous recommendation and pass it on to the full thirty-man board of trustees. Unfortunately, they won't meet again until the second half of next month." He turned to Dummer. "I suppose you don't mind staying on until then."

"I'll do anything to help," said Dummer.

For an extra three thousand dollars, said Crunch to himself, I'm sure he would. On the way out he whispered to Frank Ray,

"I wish you would get to hell out of here and go to the Bahamas."

Unfortunately Ray would not have had much time to lie on the beach. At eight in the morning five days later Scotti telephoned Jim.

"Frank had a pulmonary hemorrhage last night."

"Will he make it?" asked Jim.

"He will this time. How about meeting me in room nine-o-nine in an hour? He wants to see you."

They found Ray flat on his back in bed, comfortable but extremely pale. The one thousand ml. of blood which Scotti had ordered were dripping rapidly into a vein at the bend of his left elbow.

"Jim," said Ray, sitting up at once. "Congratulations. You're in like Flynn. Ratification by the board of trustees in February is a mere formality. For the first time we'll be in control of the hospital, by only four votes to three, it's true, but still in control, and of almost everything except the naming of a new director. The only question is what will happen when I am no longer around."

There was a gentle tap on the door. Jenny Velvet walked in on her toes like a beautiful ballet dancer afraid of waking the audience. Clutched to her abdomen was a stenographer's notebook, the attached pencil pointing upward to one seductively outlined breast. Dropping to her knees by the bedside, she kissed the palm of his left hand gently without interrupting the flow of blood which was dripping through the plastic tubing.

"I came as soon as I heard," she said. "Can I take down any last words? Any last instructions?" Mistaking his look of consternation for one of concern for her, she cried, "It's no trouble, no trouble at all. I can take everything down in shorthand, rush back to my office, type it all up, and have it back here in time for you to sign while you're still able."

She kissed his hand again and a dreamy look came into her eyes. "Whenever your wife went away, I always wanted to spend the night with you. Oh, I knew you were sick. I would never have let it get too exciting. And afterwards, I would have taken care of you."

Frank Ray smiled. "Jenny, Jenny, I'm not going to die this time. This is just a dress rehearsal."

She blushed. "If I had known that, I would never have said those things about going to bed with you."

"Don't feel bad, Jenny. It was a great compliment."

"I didn't mean it that way," she said. "I meant that now that you know you could have had me, you will be sad because of all the fun you missed." She hesitated and then added philosophically, "But there's a heaven and we'll both be there."

Frank laughed. "The question is, will you love me in the next world as you did in this?"

"More. You won't be sick anymore, and I'll make love to you until your ears ring."

He smiled, lay back again, and closed his eyes. Jenny kissed his hand for the third time and tiptoed out of the room. As soon as he heard the door close, he opened his eyes.

"I've got to hand it to you, Frank," said Scotti. "You haven't lost your sex appeal. All that radiation hasn't damaged your balls."

"I only wish my lungs were as good," said Frank. He sat up. "Let's get down to business. I'm not going to last forever. When I go, the medical board will be split down the middle, three votes to three, you two and Airov against the old gang, Bligh, Grant, and Akt. The man who takes my place will cast the crucial vote. Our three opponents will try to bring in some kid from the outside whom they can lead around by the nose. The logical man for the job is my assistant and right arm, good old Haynes, who has worked for Adams for twenty years. Not only will he run a good department, he will vote the way I would have."

"No argument," said Scotti, "but on a three-to-three vote how is he going to get in?"

Ray turned to Jim. "It's up to you. You will have to violate a sacred tabu which states that a doctor must never bypass the medical board, never go directly to the trustees to sell them a bill of goods. We call it an end run. You will be pulling a fast one, but you will have to go directly to Guthrie and Crunch for that fourth vote. They owe you a lot. You've got them by the short hairs."

"I'll go," said Jim.

Ray gave a sigh of relief. "That's all I wanted to hear."

"Don't let this hemorrhage get you down," said Jim. "Nobody expected the virus killer to pop up the way it did. One morning you'll read in the *New York Times* that the Mayo Clinic, or Harvard, or Memorial, or Johns Hopkins, or the Medical Center, or most likely Rockefeller has invented something just as good for your condition."

"Frank," said Scotti, "I have a hunch that when you are ninety we will have to take you out in the backyard and shoot you."

Ray smiled, lay back, and closed his eyes. "Thanks."

Jeez, said Jim to himself, he's as pale as the sheet. I wish the blood would run in faster.

In the corridor he and Scotti saw Mrs. Ray coming toward them with a bunch of bright red roses in her hands. She was thin and pale, and her shoulders drooped. When she reached the door, she gave them a small, defeated smile and said apologetically,

"Roses for Frank's cheeks."

20

AT NINE THIRTY on the morning of February twentieth 1974 a notice appeared on every bulletin board in John Quincy Adams Hospital announcing that Dr. James Keats had been appointed Director of Pediatrics. At eleven o'clock his lawyer telephoned him that Annie Laurie had obtained her divorce and that Wells had married her the next day. At twelve thirty he walked into Trudy Starr's office looking as if he had just scored the winning touchdown in the Rose Bowl.

"I know, I know, Herr Direktor," she said, feeling as if she were a young supervisor in Heidelberg once more. "Congratulations. You will never be a loser again."

"That's only the shrimp cocktail. Wait until you hear about the main course. I'm free. And Wells has married Annie Laurie."

She laughed. "I'm going to write to my congressman to have February twentieth declared a national holiday."

"It's officially celebrated tonight. Where would you like to go? To the Waldorf again?" He made it sound as if they went there twice a week.

"I'd like to go to a quiet and very exclusive French restaurant."

"There's La Femme Dorée. It's so exclusive that once, so I was told, they turned away J. Pierpont Morgan, then the most powerful financier in the world, because of his bulbous red nose. They claimed it showed he was an alcoholic. He had to bring a letter from his physician testifying that he had acne rosacea before they would let him in."

"Oh, certainly. He would have bought out the place and everyone in it and sold them off into slavery for their impudence. But I would love to go, Jimmy."

He patted her awkwardly on the arm. "I'll be back at two thirty for grand rounds. Later in the afternoon I have appointments set up at the Medical Center with Professor Choate and Professor Locke. Those two interviews could make or break me."

"It will be a breeze. Locke and Choate will welcome you to the club. But don't invite them for dinner."

In the main lobby on the way out he met Dummer.

"Congratulations, but I don't envy you," said the man he had just replaced. "You are in the same spot I was in before I got Wells. Wait until you see how hard it is to run a department without residents and without the benevolent interest of the Medical Center."

"I'm not going to wait," said Jim.

At two twenty-five he returned to the pediatric floor, where fourteen residents and three nurses were standing in freshly pressed uniforms. He nodded to them and walked into Trudy Starr's office.

She rose and said, "Put on a show, Jimmy. Let these kids see what the old man can do."

"I might at that," he said.

Then he followed her back to the floor and addressed himself to the residents. "This is the last grand rounds that I will conduct under the old system. I am handing the Department of Pediatrics back to the doctors. When I make grand rounds again, I will be accompanied not only by you but by all the attendings. On every other day of the week a senior attending and two of lesser rank will make their own rounds. You will be surprised to learn how much they can teach you at the bedside. This service has been run by a general and a lot of privates. The time has come for the other officers to move in."

He turned to the chief resident. The young doctor had a beard and shoulder-length hair, thus combining the cephalic attributes of an Edwardian professor of medicine with those of a King Arthur page boy.

"There are forty beds on this floor," said Jim. "How many patients do you have?"

The young man seemed startled. "I don't know, sir."

"Miss Starr, do you know?" asked Jim.

"Twenty-eight," said Trudy.

"And, Doctor, how many of those are on the pediatric service?" asked Jim. "Please don't puff up your census by including the children on the surgical, ear-nose-and-throat, orthopedic, and eye services."

The chief resident seemed embarrassed. "I don't know, sir."

"Miss Starr?" asked Jim.

"There are fourteen patients on the pediatric service."

"Fourteen patients and fourteen residents," said Jim. "I'm glad to see that you are not outnumbered. And of the fourteen patients I don't suppose you know how many are taken care of by their own private doctors and how many are on the ward."

The chief resident shook his head. Surprisingly, his long hair did not swirl.

"There are five ward patients," said Trudy. "The rest are private and semiprivate patients."

"I can see," said Jim to the house staff, "that you are neither outnumbered nor overworked."

The residents who had spent so much of their day away from the floor that they were not familiar with the cases stirred uneasily. Aware of this and of his own lack of preparation, the chief resident said,

"Things are very slow, sir. There's really not much to show. Would you care to go to the small conference room with us and tell us how you want the service run?"

"Some other day," said Jim. "Now I want to see a couple of patients."

He turned into a room where a thirteen-year-old blue-eyed boy was staring at the ceiling, his skin the color of the half-milk half-coffee concoction that indulgent parents sometimes let their little children have.

"He's an old rheumatic," said the chief resident without much enthusiasm, "with heart involvement but no joint manifestations. For some reason his fever won't respond to aspirin or salicylates."

He held up the chart to demonstrate the spiking temperature curve.

Jim made no attempt to examine the boy. Instead, he lifted the sheet from the foot of the bed and pinched his big toenail. The patient screamed. Everyone froze. Jim patted him gently on the head, said, "I'm sorry," and walked out.

He turned to the house staff. "That boy doesn't have rheumatic fever. He has SBE, subacute bacterial endocarditis, with clusters of bacteria on the valves and lining of his heart."

"We've done three blood cultures and they are all negative," protested the chief resident.

"Do three more. Eventually you will pick up the causative organism. If it is streptococcus viridans, and I think it is, you can save his life with massive doses of penicillin. Get moving before it's too late."

"I took a fourth culture two days ago," said José. "It might be ready now."

Trudy pointed her finger and one of the nurses hurried to the telephone. Jim and his entourage walked slowly along the corridor. In a moment the young girl returned with a piece of paper which she handed to José.

"Streptococcus viridans," he read.

The residents were stunned.

"How were you able to make the diagnosis, sir, without examining the patient?" said one who looked like a well-fed baby behind his mutton-chop whiskers and walrus mustache.

"It's not a method I recommend," said Jim, "but this is the way it's done. First, when did you ever hear of an uncomplicated case of rheumatic fever that did not respond to aspirin or salicylate? Second, look at the boy's complexion. He has the typical café-au-lait color of SBE. Third, and this is not well known, SBE sometimes causes exquisitely tender subungual hemorrhages, especially under the nail of the big toe. I can see that you are wondering how I was able to guess the organism. Well, eighty percent of cases of SBE in children are caused by strep viridans."

He took a few steps ahead and then turned around. "There is an art of medicine and a science of medicine. When the chief shows off, that's called the fun of medicine."

The fourteen residents relaxed.

"If the chief resident doesn't object, I would like to show you one more case," said José, "but I must warn you that it will make you sad."

"I've seen sick children before. Why should it make me sad?" asked Jim.

"Because you could save this little girl's life if you had the virus killer. Since it's all gone, she's doomed, I'm afraid. This time, sir, you are going into the bull ring with nothing but your hands. Even Belmonte needed the muleta and the sword."

"It's better than walking away," said Jim.

"I hope you will not think me presumptuous, sir," said José, "but I went to the record room and read through Charlie Prince's chart. He is the police captain's son with the Guillain Barré Syndrome whose life you saved with the virus killer. This case is a replica."

Trudy handed him the patient's chart. "Four days ago this ten-year-old girl flew up from Louisiana with her parents," he continued. "She had mild diarrhea, but so did many of the people in the little town where she lived. We think the diarrhea was caused by an intestinal virus. Three days ago her temperature rose to one hundred and two and she complained of dizziness, nausea, and weakness of her feet. Two days ago both legs became paralyzed and she was admitted to Adams."

"What was her blood count?" asked Jim.

"Low, a typical viral count," answered José. He paused. "Her knee jerks were absent. The paralysis ascended rapidly, just as it did with Charlie Prince. Yesterday it reached her abdominal muscles and her upper extremities; today, her pharynx. She can't swallow. We expect her respiratory muscles to become paralyzed next. We have the respirator by her bedside."

"And your diagnosis?" asked Jim.

"Dr. Dummer and the house staff feel she has the Guillain Barré Syndrome caused by an intestinal virus, just like Charlie Prince," answered José. He looked mournful. "The worst part is that we can't do anything for her. She was such a trusting and brave little girl. Just before she lapsed into a stupor, she made me promise that I would show her New York." He looked through the doorway at the patient. "I know a doctor should not be sentimental, but she reminds me of Ravel's Pavane from *The Death of an Infanta*."

"So she should. It was written about a dying Spanish princess. And don't worry about being sentimental. It has at least one advantage. Nobody will mistake you for a hospital administrator." Jim smiled. "The best football player I ever came across was a sentimental middle linebacker. Before every game he would send his invalid mother a bunch of roses. Then he would go out on the field and take the opposing quarterback apart."

He reached for the chart and read the history. "What did the spinal fluid show?"

"Nothing," answered José. "It was perfectly normal."

Jim frowned and shook his head. "I think the town she lived in is in a wooded area," he added with seeming irrelevance.

Then he walked to the bedside, followed by his retinue.

The big Bennett respirator stood in the center of the room like a lifeguard on a beach. A frail, little, dark-haired girl lay semiconscious on her back, drooling because her swallowing muscles were paralyzed.

"It would take only three ml. of the virus killer to save her," said José.

Jim looked grim. "You can't practice medicine on vain regrets."

He performed the routine physical and neurological examinations rapidly. Then, to everyone's surprise, he went over the child's skin inch by inch. Last of all he inspected her scalp, and, after turning her on her side, the area where the base of her skull joined her neck in back. Suddenly he looked up.

"The normal spinal fluid should have tipped you off. If she had the Guillain Barré Syndrome, like Charlie Prince, the protein would have been elevated. If she had a viral encephalitis, the white cells would have been elevated."

He paused to accentuate the importance of what he was about to say. "She doesn't have a viral infection at all. She has tick paralysis."

He parted the hair at the back of her neck just below her skull. There, an inch away from her brain, clutching her skin in its devil's grip, was a dark, ugly tick smaller than a dime.

He used his flat, teaching voice. "If this were the spring and she had been bitten in Colorado, I would say that it was the Rocky Mountain wood tick, *dermacentor andersoni*. But since she just came up from Louisiana, it is probably a close relative, *dermacentor variabilis*."

He turned to Trudy. "Miss Starr, would you please get me some ether and a sterile pack with a forceps and a scalpel?"

Trudy snapped her fingers. Two nurses ran from the room.

"Children are the principal victims of tick paralysis," he went on. "The closer the bite is to the brain, the more deadly the symptoms. No virus is involved. When the tick takes its blood meal, it injects a neurotoxin, a nerve poison, into the skin, perhaps in its saliva. The venom causes a rapidly ascending, flaccid paralysis indistinguishable from that of the Guillain Barré Syndrome."

The two nurses returned out of breath. Trudy laid the instruments on a sterile towel on top of the table next to Jim.

"There are many ways to remove a tick," he said, "from touching it with a hot match to just pulling it off. Unfortunately, if you leave the mouthpart in the skin, there's trouble."

Trudy and one of the nurses turned the child on her chest. Jim poured a little ether on the tick, which lay motionless in its bed of hair, feeding on the patient.

"Some experts feel that ether may make it relax its grip," he said as he put on rubber gloves.

He grasped the body of the tick with the forceps and pulled it gently. At the same time he slipped the tip of the scalpel under the mouthpart, which was deeply imbedded in the skin. The tick came out at once. He held it up with the forceps and pointed with the scalpel.

"Everything is here, including the mouthpart. Send it up to the lab," he added as he put the tick and the instruments on the towel.

The child had not moved. He took off his gloves, applied disinfectant to the puncture, and turned her on her back.

"You didn't see the tick," he said to the residents, "because it was hidden by her hair." He patted her on the shoulder. "In a few hours there will be a marked improvement. In a few days she will be able to leave the hospital."

The baby-faced resident with the mutton-chop whiskers and the walrus mustache stood with his mouth open. He closed it slowly, waited, and then asked,

"What would have happened if you hadn't removed the tick?"

"The child would have died," Jim shot back.

A terrible silence settled over the room. He walked to the corridor, turned around, and faced his staff. No one said anything. No one knew what to say. At last José stepped forward, bowed, and said,

"We, your residents, salute you. You triumphed without the muleta and the sword."

Jim pointed through the doorway to the girl who was already beginning to stir. He turned to José and said,

"A gentleman of the old school never breaks his word. Remember, you promised to show her New York."

He walked away with Trudy at his side. When they reached the elevator, she looked up at him and said,

"You are really a competitive male. I think you put on this virtuoso performance to impress me because Backman, that other incomparable diagnostician, came here and put on one of his own, and then surveyed my figure with his connoisseur's eyes."

Jim gave her a crooked smile. "Why else?"

She squeezed his hand. "There was another reason, wasn't there, Jimmy?"

"I suppose so. I guess I did it for the old docs, the has-beens, the former greats, the ones who get their shoes half-soled because full soles cost nine dollars, the ones with the ten-thousand-dollar life-insurance policies in their bank vaults, the ones who don't have a Trudy Starr to make them young and important again."

The elevator door opened. He squeezed her hand and said, "Dress up tonight."

21

PROMPTLY AT four that afternoon Jim entered Professor Choate's office. The virologist rose at once. So did Mr. Wright, who had insisted on being present whenever Jim visited his medical-school classmate.

"Congratulations on your Adams appointment," said the old man, adding thoughtfully, "Of course, there should never have been any doubt. Now sit down and tell me in detail all about the last days of the virus killer."

Jim related the miraculous cures of Corky Guthrie and Clair Crunch, omitting only their names although he was sure that his listener knew them well.

"You marched away with the band playing and the colors flying," said the seventy-five-year-old trustee. "If Choate here had done as well with his half as you have done with yours, we would now have a Nobel Prize discovery in our hands. And to think that I have given him millions and you never a cent!"

"That shows how wise you were," said Jim. He turned to Choate. "Bill, I came here for your help. Mr. Guthrie and Mr. Crunch have each donated a quarter of a million dollars for a department of pediatric virology. Another half million dollars must be raised before it can open. I'm supposed to run it."

"We know all about it," said Choate.

"You also know that I'm no virologist. The question arises, who is going to design the unit, buy the equipment, and hire the personnel?"

Choate smiled. "We'll do it together. I'll take you under my wing. I'll be your unofficial, or if you wish your official, consultant."

"And don't worry about the other half million dollars," said Wright, "or about what Crunch and Guthrie will say. I'll take care of everything. I've been faithful to Choate's department long enough. Now I'll have an occasional roll in the hay with yours. I'll tell you this, though. The new virology department at Adams is not going to be named after Corky and Clair, as fond as I am of them. You can't have buildings named after children. Let them get married and put up one of their own. I want it named after the mad technician who created the virus killer. You know who he is, of course."

"Of course," said Choate.

"He showed the way," Wright went on. "He demonstrated that such a drug can be developed. Over a hundred years ago, Jules Verne in *Twenty Thousand Leagues Under the Sea* conceived the idea of the modern submarine. The reality did not appear until the twentieth century. Choate, your mad technician is the Jules Verne of virology. I am determined that the new department at Adams shall be known as his." He stroked his chin. "You can be sure that somewhere in this city a mother and father are trying to smile as they say, 'Doing nicely,' at the mention of his name. I trust that they will be invited to the dedication."

"Certainly, sir," said Jim. "And a suitable tribute will be paid to your generosity."

"I won't permit it," said Wright. "I am always the anonymous donor," he coughed gently, "whose name is later leaked to every newspaper in the country. My publicity department sees to that."

Jim laughed. "Thank you for your generosity both as an audience and as a philanthropist." He turned to Choate. "And thanks, Bill, for never forgetting that we were once in the same class."

Wright gave him a strange look. "More than twenty years ago I met your fiancée at one of the great houses in England. Oh, come,

come, we are both men of the world. She *is* your fiancée, isn't she? I have never forgotten her. She was incandescent, positively incandescent. I wonder whether she remembers me."

Jim smiled. "I'm sure no woman could ever forget you even if she lived to be a hundred."

Professor Choate stood up and pressed the switch on his sugar-cube-sized tape recorder. A series of tiny but incredibly clear staccato clicks filled the room.

"Don't tell me that your Nobel Prize winners have taken to talking in code," said Wright.

The six-foot-six virologist smiled and looked down benignly. "This is a proton bombardment of the atomic nucleus."

"Choate," said the old trustee, "after all these years I know you well. You've gone out and recorded a ping-pong match."

Jim said goodbye and walked up to Dr. Locke's office on the floor above.

"Sit down, Jim," said the professor of pediatrics, "I'm glad there's a desk between us this time instead of one of your blockers. Don't look so grim. You don't intend to run through me and I'm not going to tackle you. We may even be on the same team."

"That would be a relief," said Jim.

"You want a departmental affiliation, don't you?"

"That's why I'm here," said Jim.

"Then you are going to have to give up a little of your independence and make a few concessions. It won't be bad."

"A Faustian bargain, is that it?"

Locke shook his head. "No. You'll leave here with your soul intact. All we ask is to have a little to say about the running of your department. Not much, and more in principle than in practice. For one thing, we would like to have a voice in the choosing of a new director." He raised his hand. "No, no, you're completely satisfactory. You've turned out some honest research in an antiresearch hospital. I've known you since college; Choate thinks highly of you; and Mr. Wright is fascinated by you. I am talking about your successor ten years from now. But by then all your directors will be full time and Adams will come to us for advice. If you have a candidate of your own, you've got ten years to train him and make him acceptable to the medical school and the Medical Center. Fair?"

"Perfectly fair."

"We are phasing out all our part-timers and volunteers. I might want to place one or two of our private practitioners in your department."

"No suburban drones, I hope."

"No. Manhattan workers."

"Sounds good," said Jim.

"Then we always have many more applicants for residencies than we can accept. I would like to send some of the better ones to you."

Jim hesitated. "Fine, but no battalions."

Locke smiled. "No battalions." He looked hard at Jim. "There might be a black among them."

This time Jim did not hesitate. "I would rather have a fifty-hour-a-week black doctor than a thirty-hour-a-week honky M.D."

"Ah, I see you know the language. There's something else. In their final year the medical students are permitted to go to other hospitals for specialty training. It gives them a different point of view. Some are particularly interested in bedside medicine. I'm going to send them to you."

"Fine. We'll do a special job on them."

"Finally, once in a while I'm going to take you to lunch. You might want to tell me what is going on in your department, especially in your new department of virology. By the way, your friend, Choate, could help you a lot."

"Thanks for the lunches. And Bill has already promised to be my coach."

"Wells turned out to be a bit of a prick, didn't he?" said Locke.

Jim shrugged. "I'm keeping him on."

"Smart politics," said Locke. He leaned back. "We will make you a clinical professor of pediatrics. Later on we will discuss associate and assistant clinical professorships for members of your staff."

"That's very decent of you," said Jim.

Locke smiled. "It goes with the affiliation." He looked out the window. "You know, Jim, we have a big department up here. We also have the problems that go with size, monetary problems, administrative problems, research problems, assembly-line problems, educational problems. You have a simple little setup at Adams with plenty of time and a nice staff." He turned back to Jim. "You should be able to run your department with such quiet elegance and such expert attention to each patient as to make it the envy of every hospital in New York."

"I'll certainly try," said Jim.

The two big men stood up, grinned, and shook hands across the desk.

22

FROM THE Medical Center Jim drove to a florist on the upper East Side, where he sent Trudy two enormous white orchids accompanied by a card which read, "From a secret admirer." Although it was growing late he could not resist the temptation to go into the electronics shop next door for a pocket calculator, which he stuffed into his back pocket after making sure that this one did not always flash "thirteen." On the extra thirty-five thousand dollars a year Adams would give him he could afford to indulge himself, he decided. Then he went home, brushed his teeth, washed, splashed shaving lotion on his face, and put on a fresh shirt and tie. Finally, he arranged to have one of the junior attendings take care of his practice for the night.

Trudy answered the door wearing a tight-fitting black dress that revealed her body in considerable detail.

"Stop staring," she said. "You're worse than Backman. Someone just sent me these beautiful orchids. He must either be a suitor or very rich."

"I think he's both," said Jim as he took off his overcoat.

"Shall we have a drink?"

"We'd better save it for La Femme Dorée. Drinks are compulsory there. Bill Choate once told me that years ago Mr. Wright tried to explain to the owner that while he liked the restaurant very much, he was unable to drink cocktails or wine for reasons of health. The proprietor stated flatly that he would have to drink both if he wanted to eat at La Femme Dorée. The next few minutes were touch and go. Finally a compromise was reached. Thirty-five dollars would be routinely added to the old man's bill. In return he would receive a complete dispensation. He would not have to drink anything, even water."

"We'll have our drink there," said Trudy firmly.

They took a taxi to East Sixty-fourth Street. She had expected to find an intimate French restaurant. Instead, they were ushered into a spacious dining room where the tables were just within hailing distance of each other, every one an enclave of culinary elegance in a pocket of insulating air. There was no clatter of dishes, probably, Jim reasoned, because the management had devised a secret process for incorporating rubber into the chinaware. The owner's grandfather had been a French physician. Because of this the policy of the restaurant had been never to place a doctor in the worst location. The tradition was still in force. The maître d' seated them in the next-to-worst location. He did not stay to take their order. They were not important enough for that, not with the floor sagging with celebrities. After half an hour their waiter appeared wearing an expression, it seemed to Jim, similar to the one he had often seen on the faces of orderlies carrying the bedpans of dysentery patients. Trudy ordered a whiskey sour, Jim a screwdriver.

"Would monsieur like to have his screwdriver with Stolichnaya?" asked the waiter, indicating by his supercilious manner that it was time the customer tried Russian vodka.

"I'd prefer to have it with Solzhenitsyn," answered Jim.

The waiter shook his head. "We don't have that."

"All right," said Jim, "I'll take whatever you've got," waving his hand like a good sport to show that he would make do with second best.

While they were sipping their drinks he told Trudy of his double triumph at the Medical Center that afternoon. Their waiter pointedly ignored them for another half hour. Then he returned to their table and laid their menus in front of them as if he were playing three card Monty.

After a moment Jim said, "The only thing I can understand here is *les huitres Rockefeller*. That must mean oysters Rockefeller. Let's have that."

Trudy nodded.

Ignoramus, the waiter said to himself. He couldn't wait until I made a few suggestions. Out loud he said,

"Very good, monsieur. Next I would suggest either *l'agneau du père rouge, l'agneau de la mère bleu, cote de veau simplicissimus, entrecôte Boulanger aux ananas, homard diabolique,* or *grenouilles sans peur.*"

He announced the selections as if each were a nobleman entering the reception room of a king.

Trudy shook her head. "I don't think you're going to like this, Jimmy. You can have lamb of the red father, lamb of the blue mother, veal cutlet simplicissimus, whatever that is, a Boulanger steak with pineapple, which sounds disgusting, a diabolical lobster, or fearless frogs."

"I want a big steak, medium rare, with French fries," Jim bellowed.

The waiter looked at him with distaste. The man was a beast. The woman probably threw him raw horsemeat once a day at home. But he was enormous, mean, and undoubtedly dangerous.

"I, too," said Trudy.

"Ah, a chateaubriand," said the waiter, "an excellent choice. As for the wine, monsieur, I think you will find our cellar adequate. I would suggest either a Chateau LaFite Rothschild 1969 or a Chateau Neuf du Pape 1963."

Jim leaned toward him and said with a conspiratorial air, "You wouldn't have a Doctor Pepper, would you?"

The waiter stiffened. I must control myself, he kept saying over and over again to himself. This madman could turn violent at any moment.

"No, monsieur, nothing like that."

"Then we'll have the Chateau LaFite Rothschild," said Jim.

The food was superb. After the busboy had cleared away the dishes, the waiter said,

"May I suggest *Pfannkuchen nach Pariser Art flambée?*"

"That must be hybrid Franco-German crepes suzette," said Trudy. "I will just have coffee."

Jim nodded that he would have the same.

"In that case I would like to inform you," said the waiter, rubbing his hands, "that we have a few rare pre-World War I cordials. May I bring you a chartreuse?"

Jim nodded again. After the man was out of earshot, he explained, "If I had said no, he would have become hysterical." He smiled at her. "Mr. Wright told me this afternoon that he had met you in England twenty years ago. He wondered if you remembered him."

She stared into the past. It must have been at one of the great houses of England to which she had been invited at the suggestion of John Gloucester. It seemed as if she had been to all of them, so vast was the power of her once-a-week lover. He had provided everything, the car, the chauffeur, the glittering social life, everything but the escort. She thought back to the top-secret Wednesday-night assignations kept regularly for seven years, to the iron rule that decreed that they must never be seen together not so much to avoid hurting his wife as to avoid damaging his career, to the picture that always came on her birthday, and to the one date that they had had together, that day at Schwetzingen when he had walked along the paths of the ducal estate ten feet away from her so that if he should come upon an acquaintance, he could pretend that he did not know her. He had been about as old then as Jimmy was now. And so slim, so exquisitely dressed, so handsome, so utterly charming, so rich, so powerful. But he had never saved a life, she was sure. And he would never have had dinner with her in a restaurant like La Femme Dorée, as the man opposite her was doing tonight.

She heard Jim ask, "Do you remember him?"

She focused on him again. "I remember him well."

The waiter hurried to the table with the chartreuse. The service was improving. Tip time was approaching. Trudy sipped the drink.

"How do you like the pre-World War I chartreuse?" asked Jim.

She shrugged. "It tastes like anything that's over fifty years old." She smiled. "Except you."

"My father used to like a song Guy Empey wrote during World War I. It was called 'Your Lips Are No Man's Land But Mine.'" He reached out and touched her lips with his fingertips. "Is it a contract?"

"Oh, Jimmy, who would want to kiss a woman of my age!"

"Any man who ever loved a beautiful wife."

They leaned across the table and kissed each other.

"It's a contract," she said.

"When I was a child, I thought that if you kissed a girl you had to marry her. I feel that way again tonight. Will you marry me, Trudy? It will be a platonic relationship, but we'll make a go of it."

"Get the check, Jimmy."

"What's the matter? Don't you like it here?"

"Let's go home, dear, and have a platonic relationship."

He signaled for the bill. It was detailed and lengthy, resembling, in fact, the yearly statements that banks send to stockholders and depositors. Everything was itemized. There was a separate charge for the bread, the butter, the water, which must have been bottled, and the use of the napkins and the tablecloth. He was lucky, he decided, that he had not spilled anything. He reached into his back pocket for the calculator and laid it on the table. With the nonchalance of a supermarket checker he tapped the keys, referring from time to time to the bill in front of him. People began to stare. One old man with a hearing aid said a trifle too loudly, "Martha, I wish I had that fellow's nerve."

When the tabulation was completed, Jim laid some large bills on the table and said, "Keep it."

The waiter bowed low. "You are very kind, sir."

Jim smiled. "It's to make up for the mockery."

The trip home in the taxi was made in silence. As soon as they entered her apartment and hung up their coats, she unpinned her orchids and put them in the refrigerator. Then she returned to the living room, turned off all the lights but one, and began to take off her dress.

"Trudy, what are you doing!" exclaimed Jim.

"I am taking off my clothes, and if you are a gentleman, you will take off yours."

He followed her into the darkened bedroom, groped for a chair, sat down, and began to untie his shoelaces.

"It's no good, Trudy. I've lost my sexual reflexes." After a moment he added gravely, "There's a chance that it might work, I suppose, if we performed fellatio and cunnilingus."

She glanced at his outline, smiled, and said, "Come to bed, Jimmy. Let's make love in English."

He lay down beside her. At first, clumsiness and panic took hold of him, but, enveloped in her warmth and compassion, his confidence blossomed. He penetrated her body with ease, and when the climax

256

came they shared it together. They knew at once exactly what they were going to say. Instead, they fell asleep in each other's arms.

At a quarter after six, the alarm rang. Jim sat up and shouted, "What's going on here!"

She turned off the buzzer, put her finger on his lips, and said, "I have a date with you at Adams at a quarter to eight. Remember?"

"You have a date with me now."

This time they came together with the assurance of old lovers.

After it was over he lay next to her and said, "You *will* marry me, won't you?"

She sighed. "I don't know, Jimmy, I don't know. The man I marry can't be slim, handsome, and rapierlike. He has to be big, mean-looking, and a little ugly."

He sat up. The sheet slid down from his huge, hairy chest.

"Look at me. I'm practically a gorilla."

She nodded. "And he can't be fastidious and wear elegant clothes."

He lay down again. "I haven't told you yet, but I am going to be nominated as one of the ten worst-dressed men of the year."

She looked into the distance. "I have to go back to Schwetzingen. Please don't ask me why. And my husband will have to take me there."

"We'll go as soon as I can get the marriage license."

"No, no, in June, when the white lilacs bloom and everybody eats white asparagus. We'll stay in Heidelberg at the Europaischer Hof and walk through the lobby trying to make ourselves conspicuous. And if any man looks at me, you'll glare at him and make a scene."

Jim showed her his big fists. "I'll give him a shot in the labonza."

"Then we'll take the streetcar that runs through the fields all the way to Schwetzingen. And you'll put your arm around me, talk in a loud voice, and make all the passengers look at us."

"I'll tell them how we beat Georgia when Sinkewich was their all-American back."

"And when we reach the ducal estate, you won't walk ten feet away from me, will you? We'll walk side by side."

"We'll be so close that people will think we're stuck together with epoxy glue."

"And I will show you the little palace where the duke's mistress once lived and the fields around it which the jealous wife had planted with onions. Only this time I'll enjoy it, because I'll be a wife, not a mistress."

"You certainly will be," he said gravely.

"Next we will stroll hand in hand to the statue of the big white stallion. Only you won't take me behind it so that nobody can see us, and pop a mint into your mouth before you kiss me. We'll just walk up the hill a little, and there in the sunlight in front of a hundred Germans you'll take me in your arms and tell me that you love me."

"I promise it, Trudy."

"Then you'll stand there with the biggest erection in Germany, sweat a little, and worry about your reflexes."

"You know me well."

"We'll each eat two plates of white asparagus, and then take the trolley back to Heidelberg. That night at the Europaischer Hof you'll make love to me again even though the bed squeaks and the people in the room below keep banging on the pipes."

"I will, and I'll try to make you forget about the other time."

She kissed him on the lips. "Of course I'll marry you."

She slid out of bed and walked to the shower. She was smiling but her eyes were moist.

Three weeks later she received a telephone call from Mr. Wright. He asked her to have tea with him that Saturday afternoon.

"Please be prompt, my dear," he said.

"I'll meet you downstairs," said Trudy.

He called for her in a big, twenty-year-old Rolls Royce driven by a seventy-year-old chauffeur with twenty/twenty vision. The new models the tycoon regarded as compacts. The car had been completely renovated. Automatic transmission, power steering, power brakes, and a new motor had been installed. The original fur lap-robes still hung from racks on the side doors but they were now reinforced by a modern heating system. And air conditioning was there as well. They went to La Femme Dorée. This time she found herself at the center table with three waiters in constant attendance. No one asked them what they wanted to drink. And no water glasses were placed before them. He talked about the Medical Center and the role of the philanthropist in the development of virology; she about the England and Germany of a generation ago.

"I met you at dinner in London twenty years ago," he said. "I was curious to find out if you had changed."

"And have I?"

"A little. My wife had died the month before." He thought back. "It was a distinguished gathering. The prime minister was there. I don't suppose you remember."

"I remember it," said Trudy, "but not because the prime minister was there. I remember it because you came over to me and said that I was as beautiful as your wife had been when she was young and the most beautiful girl in the world."

"You have a kind memory." He took a sip of his tea. "I am going to do a little fishing. Do you intend to invite me to the wedding?"

"I do now," said Trudy.

"Are your parents alive?"

"They died before I went to England."

"Uncles, brothers, a very old friend?"

She shook her head.

"Somebody has to walk down the aisle with you," said the old man. "May I ask for the privilege? My daughter would have been your age. She died when she was twenty of an overwhelming viral infection, a viral encephalitis, two weeks after we announced her engagement. She looked just like her mother."

"I'd love to have you give me away," said Trudy. "Then I won't feel deserted when I walk toward the altar and Jim."

"Thank you. The choice of a wedding present is never easy. Would you and Dr. Keats like a picture?"

Trudy threw up her hands. "Anything but that. Will you let me show you why? It will be good for me because I have never discussed my collection with anyone before."

They drove to her apartment at once. She went from picture to picture with him, telling him everything she knew about each.

"I am honored to have been selected for this once-in-a-lifetime tour," he said. "And by so charming a guide. I see that they are all scenes of England." He gave her a shrewd look. "You were a friend of John Gloucester's, weren't you?"

"Yes. And I don't want to add to his collection or start another. If Jim ever asks me how I got them, I will tell him. And then either sell them or donate them to a museum in England."

"Sell them," said the financier. "And do it even if he doesn't ask."

Early in May she sent her resignation to the nursing office. The hospital gave her a farewell tea which almost everyone attended, including the trustee members of the joint conference committee. When Hexter presented her with a silver tea service, he unbent enough to say,

"Again we lose our incomparable Pediatric Nursing Supervisor. Only this time we will gain a director's wife."

She held the wedding reception at the Carlyle. From the Medical Center came the Choates and the Lockes; from Adams, the Airovs, the Scottis, and the Rays. The radiologist looked surprisingly well. He had not yet had another pulmonary hemorrhage. She could hear the Crunches and the Guthries scolding him for not taking time off. Mr. Wright came up to her just before he left and handed her an envelope.

"Your wedding present," he said with a courtly bow.

"It's like the Academy Awards," she said as she took out the check.

It was made out to the James and Trudy Keats Fund for the Study of Anti-Viral Substances, in the amount of two hundred and fifty thousand dollars.

She threw her arms around him and kissed him on the lips.

"I can see," he said, "that I will have to enlarge my philanthropy portfolio to include projects which involve beautiful and responsive women."

Jim waited until he left. Then he came over to her and said,

"What happened to our contract? It was supposed to be 'Your Lips Are No Man's Land But Mine.' You've only been married a couple of hours and already you're carrying on with other men."

"Oh, Jimmy, he's seventy-five."

She handed him the check. She could see that he was pleased, but all he said was,

"At a quarter of a million dollars a kiss, how many will I be able to afford?"

Their month-long honeymoon in Europe was a triumph over the past. They returned to Schwetzingen twice.

One afternoon in July, while looking for a larger apartment near the hospital, Trudy came face to face with Annie Laurie. There was a long, quiet moment. Noticing that her features were already thickened, Trudy asked,

"How is your pregnancy coming along?"

"As smooth as silk. It's too bad it couldn't have happened long ago and frequently."

There was another long pause.

"And how is Dr. Wells?" asked Trudy politely.

Annie Laurie shook her head slowly in exasperation. "He's put on fifteen pounds around the middle and snores his head off every night. He's getting to be as bad as Jim."

"Oh, Jim doesn't snore anymore," said Trudy pleasantly. "It all depends on whom he sleeps with."

She smiled, inclined her head, and walked briskly away. But only because she was in a hurry. She had invited the Scottis, the Airovs, and the Rays for dinner that evening to celebrate the three months' vacation the radiologist had at last promised to take.

Everyone came on time. No one commented on the pale patches that stood out so conspicuously on the walls. Early that morning she had sent her pictures to the Parke Bernet Gallery to be sold at auction. As the four directors and their wives sat down at the table, Scotti said,

"Old football buddy, you're riding the crest of the wave. You have Trudy, your directorship," here he glanced at the squares and rectangles that were everywhere on the walls, "and money. What else do you want?"

Jim gave him a level stare. "Ten years and ten quarts of the virus killer."

Trudy touched his hand and prayed that God would give him more.